Kirby I. Bland • Michael G. Sarr
Markus W. Büchler • Attila Csendes
Oliver James Garden • John Wong
Editors

Critical Care Surgery

Handbooks in General Surgery

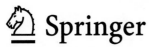 Springer

Editors

Kirby I. Bland, MD
Fay Fletcher Kerner Professor
and Chairman
Department of Surgery
Deputy Director,
Comprehensive Cancer Center
University of Alabama School
of Medicine
Birmingham, AL, USA

Markus W. Büchler, MD
Professor of Surgery and
Chairman
Department of General and
Visceral Surgery
University of Heidelberg
Heidelberg, Germany

Attila Csendes, MD, FACS (Hon)
Professor of Surgery and
Chairman
Department of Surgery
University Hospital
Santiago, Chile

Michael G. Sarr, MD
James C. Mason Professor of
Surgery
Department of Surgery
Mayo Clinic College of
Medicine
Rochester, MN, USA

O. James Garden, MBChB, MD,
FRCS (Ed), FRCP (Ed),
FRACS (Hon)
Regius Professor of Clinical
Surgery
Department of Clinical and
Surgical Sciences
The University of Edinburgh
Royal Infirmary of Edinburgh
Edinburgh, UK

John Wong, BSc (Med (Syd)),
MBBS
(Syd), PhD (Syd), MD (Hon
(Syd)), FRACS, FRCS (Edin),
FRCS (Glasg), FACS (Hon)
Chair Professor
Department of Surgery
The University of Hong Kong
Queen Mary Hospital
Hong Kong, China

ISBN 978-1-84996-377-0   e-ISBN 978-1-84996-378-7

DOI 10.1007/978-1-84996-378-7

Springer London Dordrecht Heidelberg New York

British Library Cataloguing in Publication Data

A catalogue record for this book is available from the British Library

Library of Congress Control Number: 2010937965

Printed on acid-free paper

Springer is part of Springer Science+Business Media (www.springer.com)

Preface

The editors designed the original textbook, *General Surgery: Principles and International Practice*, from which this shorter paperback monograph on critical care surgery was taken to be an accessible, concise, and state-of-the-art volume that explores and documents evolutionary principles in the practice of surgery. This work is aimed at the general surgeon and the resident in training. The scientific community continues to witness extraordinary advances in the therapy of both benign and malignant surgical diseases of various organ sites. Much of this progress has been evident over the past decade with new concepts and techniques of management that allow the surgeon to integrate this discipline with medicine, pharmacology, immunology, biostatistics, pathology, genetics, medical and radiation oncology, and diagnostic radiology and imaging. Further, each of these major disciplines contributes a small component for the diagnostic and therapeutic approaches to clinical care; hence the comprehensive planning, integration, and provision of patient care throughout the preoperative, intraoperative, and postoperative phases of care remains essential in the successful practice of our specialty.

The editors acknowledge that the aim of this work is to provide an illustrative, instructive, and comprehensive review that depicts the rationale of basic operative principles essential to surgical therapy. In organizing this monograph, the editors chose authors renowned in the disciplines for illustrating, forming, and depicting in a comprehensive fashion the surgical therapy expectant for metabolic, infectious, endocrine, and neoplastic abnormalities in adult and pediatric patients **from a truly international and multi-continental perspective.** The editors and authors were chosen carefully from across geographies and also from multi-cultural and diverse locations. While the authors consider this text to be inclusive regarding the technical and operative conditions for perioperative care in this field, its purpose should not be intended to replace standard textbooks of surgery nor should it be considered complete in its coverage of pathophysiologic disorders. In contrast, this monograph is organized to familiarize practicing surgeons, residents, and fellows with state-of-the-art surgical principles and techniques essential to contemporary practice. Therefore, the tenor of this monograph on critical care surgery has been developed to coexist with other major surgical reference texts that are dedicated—some in more comprehensive fashion—to the therapy of individual organs of systemic diseases. This monograph is much more a "working text" for the practicing surgeon with emphasis on diagnosis and treatment of critical illness. Along with this monograph, nine other paperback monographs are available and focus on the general principles of surgery, trauma, esophagus and stomach, small bowel, colorectal, liver and biliary, pancreas and spleen, oncology, and endocrine organs, all adapted from the primary textbook—*General Surgery: International Principles and Practice.*

The chapters in this monograph on critical care surgery include a condensed bibliography of highly selective journal articles, reviews, and text. In this manner of attempting to be concise, we hope to provide a precise focus for the education of the reader relative to accepted surgical principles involved in patient care. Moreover, the editors have sought to provide a counterpoint view for the selection of therapy by presenting at the opening of each chapter a list of "Pearls and Pitfalls" that highlight particular concerns or controversies. The chapters provide pertinent, though not exhaustive, summaries of anatomy and physiology, a history of surgical illness, and stages of operative approaches with relevant technical considerations outlined in an easily understandable manner.

Complications are reviewed when appropriate for the organ system, diseases, and problem. The text is supported amply by line drawings and photographs that depict anatomic or technical principles. The editors have made every attempt to minimize duplicative or repetitive discussions except when controversial or state-of-the-art issues are presented. Moreover, the editors have attempted to ensure that accurate presentations and illustrations depict properly the most complex problems confronted by the general surgeon.

Finally, in an attempt to address advances in contemporary concepts, the text has been organized to address in detail expeditious, safe, and anatomically accurate operations and incorporate standard as well as evolving surgical principles and techniques. These principles have been tested in the clinics of valid scientific knowledge and are well supported by the time-tested approaches that have been provided by practicing surgeons. The editors are excited to be able to respond to the challenge of developing a truly international text and are indeed hopeful that our readers will find this focused monograph on critical care surgery to be a repository of insight, useful, and timely information.

Kirby I. Bland
Michael G. Sarr
Markus W. Büchler
Attila Csendes
O. James Garden
John Wong

Contents

Contributors

Paul E. Bankey, MD, PhD
Director of the Trauma Institute and Associate Professor
of Surgery, Department of Surgery, University of Rochester
Medical Center, Rochester, NY, USA

Philip S. Barie, MD, MBA, FCCM, FACS
Professor of Surgery and Public Health, Department
of Surgery and Public Health, Weill Medical College of
Cornell University, New York, NY, USA

L. D. Britt, MD, MPH, FACS
Chairman Brickhouse Professor of Surgery,
Department of Surgery, Eastern Virginia Medical School
Norfolk, VA, USA

Rebecca C. Britt, MD
Assistant Professor, Department of Surgery, Eastern Virginia
Medical School, Norfolk, VA, USA

Ayesha S. Bryant, MSPH, MD
Assistant Professor, Division of Cardiothoracic Surgery,
Department of Surgery, University of Alabama
at Birmingham, Birmingham, AL, USA

Gordon L. Carlson, BSc, MBChB, MD, FRCS
Professor, Department of Surgery, University of Manchester,
Hope Hospital, Manchester, UK

Paul M. Dark, BSc, MBChB, PhD, FCEM, FRCS
Senior Lecturer, Intensive Care Department, Hope Hospital,
University of Manchester, Manchester, UK

Clifford S. Deutschman, MS, MD, FCCM
Professor of Surgery, Department of Anesthesiology
& Critical Care, University of Pennsylvania School of
Medicine, Philadelphia, PA, USA

Soumitra R. Eachempati, MD, FACS
Associate Professor of Surgery and Public Health,
Department of Surgery and Public Health, Weill Medical
College of Cornell University, New York, NY, USA

M. Sean Grady, MD
Charles Harrison Frazier Professor, Department
of Neurosurgery, University of Pennsylvania,
Philadelphia, PA, USA

James W. Jones, MD, PhD
Visiting Professor of Medical Ethics, Center for Medical
Ethics and Health Policy, Baylor College of Medicine,
Houston, TX, USA

Patrick K. Kim, MD
Assistant Professor, Department of Surgery,
University of Pennsylvania School of Medicine Trauma
Center at Penn, Philadelphia, PA, USA

James K. Kirklin, MD
Professor & Director, Division of Cardiothoracic Surgery,
Department of Surgery, University of Alabama
at Birmingham, Birmingham, AL, USA

Lorrie A. Langdale, MD
Associate Professor, Department of Surgery,
University of Washington and VA - Puget Sound Health
Care, Seattle, WA, USA

Joshua M. Levine, MD
Assistant Professor Co-Director, Neurocritical Care
Program, Department of Neurology, University
of Pennsylvania, Philadelphia, PA, USA

James M. Markert, MD, MPH
Professor and Director, Division of Neurosurgery,
Department of Surgery, University of Alabama
at Birmingham, Birmingham, AL, USA

John C. Marshall, MD, FRCSC, FACS
Professor of Surgery, Departments of Surgery & Critical
Care Medicine, St. Michael's Hospital, Toronto, Canada

Laurence B. McCullough, PhD
Professor of Medicine and Medical Ethics, Associate
Director for Education Center for Medical Ethics and
Health Policy, Baylor College of Medicine, Houston, TX,
USA

Lisa K. McIntyre, MD
Assistant Professor, Department of General Surgery,
Harborview Medical Center, Seattle, WA, USA

Lena M. Napolitano, MD, FACS, FCCP, FCCM
Professor, Department of Surgery and Surgical Critical Care,
University of Michigan Health System, Ann Arbor, MI, USA

Mamerhi O. Okor, MD
Assistant Professor, Division of Neurosurgery, Department
of Surgery, University of Alabama at Birmingham,
Birmingham, AL, USA

Priya Sampathkumar, MD
Consultant, Division of Infectious Diseases, Mayo Clinic
College of Medicine, Rochester, MN, USA

Martin D. Smith, MBBCh(Wits), FCS(SA)
Adjunct Professor, Department of Surgery, Chris Hani
Baragwanath Hospital, University of the Witwatersrand,
Johannesburg, South Africa

Jacobus S. Vermaak, MBBCh(Wits)
Department of Surgery, Chris Hani Baragwanath Hospital,
University of the Witwatersrand, Johannesburg, South Africa

1
Acute Renal Failure

Paul E. Bankey

Pearls and Pitfalls

- Post-operative acute renal failure (ARF) is often linked to the diagnosis and resolution of an evolving complication. An aggressive approach to potentially surgically correctable complications causing ARF is warranted.
- An anastomotic leak or intraabdominal abscess can cause ARF with or without systemic infection and should be ruled out early in the setting of oliguria and a rising creatinine.
- Prerenal ARF results from loss of effective circulating volume without direct parenchymal damage to the kidney unless the hypoperfusion is unrecognized or under-treated resulting in progression to ATN. The initial goal in the management of the perioperative ARF is the optimization of the patient's hemodynamic and volume status and by inference renal perfusion. Aggressive volume expansion and maintenance of a MAP >70 is recommended early in the course of oliguric ARF.
- In patients who are still producing urine, a loop diuretic, such as furosemide, administered in combination with a thiazide (cortical collecting tubule) diuretic, such as hydrochlorothiazide or metolazone, may sustain and improve urine output converting oliguric ARF to high-output ARF and an improved outcome.

K.I. Bland et al. (eds.), *Critical Care Surgery*,
DOI 10.1007/978-1-84996-378-7_1,
© Springer-Verlag London Limited 2011

- Aminoglycoside nephrotoxicity occurs in a startling 5–15% of patients treated with these drugs. In the setting of concurrent risk factors it is recommended to utilize equally effective non-nephrotoxic antibiotics such as extended spectrum penicillins, cephalosporins, carbapenems, or monobactams.
- Low dose dopamine (1–3 µg/kg/min) has been used to increase renal blood flow in disease processes associated with renal vasoconstriction such as sepsis or liver failure. Recent literature suggests that this practice should be abandoned. Dopamine has not been shown to prevent nor alter the course or outcome of ARF. Dopamine has been shown to have significant adverse effects on the heart, lungs, gastrointestinal tract, endocrine, and immunologic function when the dose is increased for use as a vasopressor.
- Patients with myoglobinuria require additional specific therapy in addition to the optimization of renal perfusion and diuresis to minimize the extent of ARF. Urine output should be maintained at >150 ml/h through the initial phases of treatment to dilute and clear precipitated and free myoglobin from the tubules.
- Urine pH should be increased above7 since myoglobin precipitation is lower at alkaline pHs. The overall goal is to produce a high-output *alkaline diuresis*.
- In patients with acute abdominal compartment syndrome, therapy is directed at relieving the intra-abdominal hypertension (>25–30 mmHg). This is most readily accomplished by laparotomy. Standard medical therapy of ARF with volume loading and inotropes usually is ineffective in this setting; however, the response to abdominal decompression is usually dramatic and life-saving.
- Nutritional support in the setting of acute renal failure should have the same goals of caloric and nitrogen equilibrium as the surgical patient without ARF. Protein support should not be withheld in fear of causing uremic complications, as this will exacerbate wasting of lean body mass and vital organs.
- The primary indications for continuous renal replacement therapy for ARF patients are refractory volume overload, the need for large amounts of blood products, and intolerance to intermittent hemodialysis due tohypotension or arrhythmias.

Introduction

Acute renal failure continues to be an important factor contributing to perioperative and post-traumatic morbidity and mortality. As an isolated organ system failure, ARF has an associated mortality of 8%; however, acute renal failure (ARF) in association with septic shock and multiple organ dysfunction syndrome has a mortality that has remained significantly higher (70–80%). In most clinical series the mortality rate from ARF continues to average 50% depending on the precipitating event, severity of comorbid conditions, and number of complications. The most cost-effective intervention in acute renal failure is its *prevention*, and the most effective means of prevention are to ensure an adequate circulating intravascular volume, avoidance of nephrotoxic agents, and to rapidly treat surgically reversible contributing causes.

There is no consensus definition of acute renal failure in critically ill patients. Recently, a classification of renal dysfunction has been proposed based on serum creatinine and urine output (Table 1.1). The classification defines a continuum of kidney dysfunction from risk to injury, and finally to renal failure.

It is rare for the general surgery patient to require direct operation on the kidney, renal vasculature, or urinary tract for treatment of acute renal failure; however, it is not infrequent that deteriorating renal function is a harbinger of a perioperative complication requiring surgical management by the general surgeon.

Clinical Presentation

The incidence of ARF is reportedly 2–5% in hospitalized patients and medical intervention frequently contributes to the problem. The three most common causes of ARF are: (1) volume depletion or hypotension; (2) aminoglycoside antibiotics; and (3) radio-contrast exposure.

TABLE 1.1. Proposed classification for acute renal failure (ARF).

	GFR criteria	Urine output criteria	
Risk	Increased SCr × 1.5	UO < 0.5 ml/kg/h for 6 h	High sensitivity
	GFR decrease > 25%		
Injury	Increased SCr × 2	UO < 0.5 ml/kg/h for 12 h	High sensitivity
	GFR decrease > 50%		
Failure	Increased SCr × 3	UO < 0.3 ml/kg/h for 24 h	High specificity
	GFR decrease > 75% or	Anuria for 12 h	
	SCr > 4 mg/dl	Oliguria	
Loss	Persistent ARF for > 4 weeks		High specificity
Eskd	End stage kidney disease > 3 months		

GFR, glomerular filtration rate; Scr, serum creatinine; UO, urine output.

Glomerular filtration rate (GFR) is the most direct indicator of renal function; however, it is difficult to measure directly in clinical practice. Serum concentrations of blood urea nitrogen (BUN) and creatinine (Cr) are more commonly used to assess renal function. The serum creatinine in most instances is an excellent barometer of renal function because a steady-state relationship exists between serum creatinine and GFR. The clinical significance is that an increase in a patient's Cr from 1 to 2 mg/dl signifies a 50% reduction in GFR and from 1 to 4 mg/dl, a 75% reduction. The correlation between Cr and GFR depends upon the assumption that it is delivered to the serum from tissue at a constant rate, which is not always the case. Patients with hypercatabolic states such as trauma or sepsis and patients with diminished muscle mass have conditions that alter the rate of Cr production, reducing the correlation of their serum concentration with renal function. Nomograms are available that accurately correlate age, ideal body weight, and Cr with GFR.

Patients with ARF may be classified based on their urine output. Oliguria is defined as urine output of <0.3 ml/kg/h for 24h or <400 ml/day(> Table 16.1). This volume represents the minimum amount of urine in which a normal daily solute load of 500 mOsm can be excreted if the kidney is maximally concentrating urine to 1,200 mOsm/kg of water. Non-oliguric ARF is defined as lack of homeostasis (electrolyte imbalance or azotemia) despite >400 ml/day of urine production. High-output ARF is defined as renal insufficiency with urine outputs >1,000 ml/day and frequently are several liters per day. The clinical relevance of this classification is that non-oliguric renal failure patients have a better prognosis then oliguric or anuric failure; therefore, management should be directed at preventing progression of non-oliguric renal failure to oliguric or anuric ARF.

The etiology of acute renal failure is often divided into three categories (see Table 1.2). *Prerenal* ARF is defined as a reversible rise in serum Cr caused by renal hypoperfusion. In prerenal ARF there is no frank renal parenchymal damage and the reduction in GFR merely reflects a drop in glomerular perfusion. Restoration of renal perfusion rapidly restores GFR and normal serum Cr levels.

Renal perfusion and GFR can be maintained at moderate levels of hypovolemia largely through the actions of sympathetic stimulation and activation of the renin-angiotensin system (autoregulation). Angiotensin II activity results in constriction of the glomerular *efferent* arteriole producing increased *efferent* arteriolar resistance. This increases hydrostatic pressure in the glomerular capillary. Eventually hypoperfusion overwhelms these compensatory mechanisms resulting in progression to renal ischemia and acute tubular necrosis (ATN). The use of Non-Steroidal Anti-Inflammatory Drugs (NSAIDs), which block synthesis of prostaglandins and are frequently used in the perioperative management of pain, are particularly hazardous in the setting of prerenal

TABLE 1.2. Major causes of acute renal failure.

Prerenal	Intrarenal	Postrenal
Intravascular volume depletion	Ischemic ATN	Neoplasm
1. Hemorrhage	1. Shock	1. Prostate
2. Vomiting	(i) Septic	2. Cervix
3. Third-spacing	(ii) Cardiogenic	3. Colorectal
4. Burns	(iii) Hypovolemic	
5. Fever		
6. Diarrhea		
Decreased cardiac output	Nephrotoxic ATN	Dysfunctional bladder
1. Congestive failure	1. Aminoglycosides	1. Anticholinergic drugs
2. Pulmonary hypertension	2. Radiocontrast agents	2. Catheter obstruction
3. Myocardial ischemia	3. Myoglobinuria	3. Prostatic enlargement
	4. Hemoglobinuria	
	5. Chemotherapeutic agents	
	6. Amphotericin B	
Decreased renal perfusion with normal or high cardiac output	Glomerulonephritis	Nephrolithiasis
1. Sepsis	1. Immune complex mediated	
2. Cirrhosis	(i) Postinfectious	
	2. Vasculitis	
Drugs	Tubulointerstitial disease	Papillary necrosis
1. Nonsteriodal anti-inflammatory agents	1. Allergic interstitial nephritis	

(continued)

TABLE 1.2. (continued)

Prerenal	Intrarenal	Postrenal
2. Angiotensin converting enzyme inhibitors		
	Other vascular	Abdominal compartment syndrome
	1. Thrombotic microangiopathy	
	2. Vascular trauma	
	3. Cholesterol embolization	

hypovolemia. Another class of drugs to avoid in the setting of prerenal hypovolemia is the Angiotensin Converting Enzyme (ACE) inhibitors that block production of angiotensin II. Both of these agents interfere with glomerular autoregulatory mechanisms and may precipitate severe renal hypoperfusion and ATN.

Intrinsic or *Intrarenal* ARF reflects direct injury to the renal parenchyma. Acute Tubular Necrosis (ATN) is the most common form of intrarenal ARF and may be caused by a variety of insults such as ischemia or nephrotoxins that lead to necrosis of the tubular epithelia (Table 1.2).

In the surgical setting ATN is frequently encountered following episodes of hypotension, commonly following resuscitation of septic or hemorrhagic shock. It may also occur post-operatively; however, many factors contribute to post-operative ATN in addition to hypotension as evidenced by the observation that in 50% of cases no hypotension is documented. In severe renal hypoperfusion, renal tubular epithelial cells develop hypoxia and necrose especially in areas where metabolic rate is high (proximal tubule and the medullary thick ascending loop of Henle). Even in the presence of relatively adequate renal blood flow severe hypoxia of tubular epithelium can develop. Ischemic epithelia slough into and obstruct the tubular lumen, producing clinically diagnostic granular casts and increased tubular backpressure, exacerbating renal ischemia by further intensifying intrarenal vasoconstriction and decreasing GFR.

Ischemic ATN secondary to renal artery occlusion is a rare cause of ARF that the general surgeon encounters primarily in the setting of blunt or penetrating trauma. The diagnosis is suggested by nonvisualization of the kidney on CT evaluation or hematuria. Irreversible renal injury develops rapidly in the setting of warm ischemia and revascularization within 6 h is the treatment goal. Controversy exists regarding the role of revascularization when the diagnosis of renal artery thrombosis is made beyond 4–6 h and overall renal salvage is low (<10%); however, case reports indicate salvage in kidneys revascularized up to 12 h after injury. Endovascular approaches to renal reperfusion may improve kidney salvage rates. Furthermore, in situations where a patient's solitary kidney is at risk, harvesting, cooling, and autotransplantation has been successfully performed.

A number of pharmacologic agents frequently used or encountered in the care of surgery patients can result in nephrotoxic ATN (Table 1.2). Antimicrobial agents commonly used in surgical patients reported to cause ATN include aminoglycosides and amphotericin B. Aminoglycoside nephrotoxicity occurs in 5–15% of patients treated with these drugs. In the setting of renal insufficiency aminoglycosides also cause ototoxicity. Recognition of injury is delayed from its onset since creatinine does not begin to increase until 7–10 days later. Aminoglycoside ARF is dose-dependent and nephrotoxicity is related to the serum concentration, particularly trough levels. Clinical guidelines have been developed for the drug concentration monitoring and dosing of aminoglycosides including both peak and trough levels, typically for gentamicin. Improved understanding of the pharmacodynamics and toxicity of aminoglycoside antibiotics has resulted in the study of once-daily dosing regimens. Although studies have suggested a therapeutic advantage and possibly a decrease in toxicity with once-daily administration, these effects have been modest. Further data are needed to clarify the role of once-daily dosing in critically ill general surgery patients. Aminoglycoside nephrotoxicity is enhanced by the interaction of NSAIDs, endotoxin, cyclosporin A, and amphotericin B and electrolyte disorders such as hypercalcemia, hypomagnesemia, hypokalemia, and metabolic acidosis. Increased nephrotoxicity is also reported in patients receiving concurrent antimicrobial therapy with cephalosporins. In the setting of concurrent risk factors it is recommended to utilize equally effective non-nephrotoxic antibiotics such as extended spectrum penicillins, cephalosporins, carbapenems, or monobactams.

Amphotericin B used for systemic fungal infections causes nephrotoxicity, in most patients. It is strongly bound to cellular membranes and alters permeability. This effect on the renal tubular epithelium leads to failure of hydrogen ion excretion and urinary loss of potassium resulting in the development of a distal type of renal tubular acidosis with hypokalemia. Loss of renal function is proportional to the dose of amphotericin and irreversible renal failure occurs at high doses (>2 g). Saline loading at the time of administration may reduce toxicity. Encapsulation of amphotericin B in liposomes or complexing of the compound with other lipid carriers brings about a major reduction in toxicity and these formulations are being utilized with increasing frequency. Newer agents such as the echinocandins are available for most common fungal infections and have reduced nephrotoxicity, replacing amphotericin B as first line agents.

Another drug related form of intrarenal ARF is interstitial nephritis, which has been classically reported following methicillin use; however, it has also been observed with other antibiotics and medications (sulfamethoxazole, rifampin). Drug-induced interstitial nephritis is considered to be of allergic origin and is often associated with a skin rash and eosinophilia.

Radiocontrast-associated ARF is relatively common because of the ubiquitous use in diagnostic and interventional treatment of general surgery patients. Contrast induced ARF usually presents within 48 h of exposure with the serum Cr peaking at 3–5 days. Frequently these patients have underappreciated preexisting intrinsic renal insufficiency concurrently with other risk factors such as advanced age, diabetes mellitus, volume depletion, or a large dye load. Hospitalized patients with a serum creatinine greater than 1.5 mg/dl have up to a 30–40% incidence of renal dysfunction after intravenous or intra-arterial contrast injection. Limiting the volume of the contrast load can reduce the risk of contrast-associated ARF. The maximum dose of contrast medium that can be safely administered has traditionally been calculated according to the formula: 5ml × kg of body wt (maximum 300 ml)/ serum creatinine. The use of nonionic, low osmolal, monomeric, contrast agents have a reduced risk and can be given in larger doses. (1.5 times ionic agents) It is recommended to avoid contrast doses without a 72 h window to allow the kidney to recover. The administration of intravenous saline to insure a replete intravascular volume prior to exposure is also recommended. Prophylactic options are summarized in Table 1.3.

Myoglobinuria is a frequent cause of nephrotoxic ARF in the surgical population. Patients with crush injuries, electrical burns, necrotizing soft-tissue infections, ischemia-reperfusion syndromes such as after revascularization, or who develop compartment syndromes are at high risk for rhabdomyolysis and myoglobinuria. Myoglobin is filtered and precipitates in the renal tubules, obstructing fluid flow, while the heme-molecule causes direct toxicity to the tubular epithelium. Patients with myoglobinuria will present with dark port-wine or tea-colored urine, which may be confused with gross hematuria initially. Serum levels of creatine phosphokinase (CPK) will characteristically be high, greater than 10,000 U/ml and at times greater than 100,000 U/ml in patients with the full-blown disease.

Postrenal ARF results from obstruction of the urinary collection system at one of several levels. Obstruction is usually prolonged and bilateral to result in ARF and prognosis for recovery is dependent on the duration of obstruction. A palpable bladder on exam indicates greater than 500 ml of retained urine consistent with obstruction. In the peri-operative or post-injury patient, it is important to demonstrate that indwelling bladder catheters are patent and within the bladder.

TABLE 1.3. Prophylaxis of contrast media-induced ARF.

Accurate history	Discontinue concomitant risks	Correction of hypovolemia
Major risk factors	Potentially nephrotoxic drugs	Isotonic saline load
1. Pre-existing impairment	1. NSAIDs	Half-isotonic saline
2. Dehydration	2. Aminoglycosides	Sodium bicarbonate soln
3. Hypovolemia	3. Amphotericin B	
	4. Vancomycin	
	5. Diuretics	
	6. ACE-inhibitors	
	7. Angiotensin receptor antagonists	
Minor risk factors	Minimize risk if diagnostic or interventional procedure with contrast medium is required	Antioxidant agents
1. Advanced age	1. Low-osmolal or iso-osmolal contrast medium (iohexol, iopamidol, ioxaglate)	N-acetylcysteine pre-treatment
2. Diabetes mellitus	2. Low amount of contrast medium	
3. Congestive heart failure	3. Wait a few days between two contrast administrations if possible	

Perform alternative diagnostic procedures in high-risk patients as able.

The acute development of abdominal compartment syndrome is increasingly being recognized as a cause of ARF that requires intervention by the general surgeon. Surgical patients can develop this syndrome following large volume resuscitation, placement of intra-abdominal packing for control of hemorrhage, prolonged operation with "tight" abdominal fascial closure, and diffuse peritonitis. The diagnosis is made clinically in a patient with high peak inspiratory pressures and CO_2 retention on the ventilator, progressive oliguria, and abdominal rigidity. Bladder pressures are measured in complex cases to confirm the clinical diagnosis with >20–30 mmHg considered significant enough, to warrant abdominal decompression, although no absolute level of intra-abdominal hypertension is considered 100% diagnostic. The cause of acute renal failure in the setting of acute abdominal compartment syndrome is multifactorial and includes reduced cardiac output secondary to decreased venous return from the vena cava, increased pressure on the renal parenchyma causing reduced renal blood flow, and increased renal venous pressure.

Diagnostic Evaluation

The evaluation of the patient with ARF has two major goals: to determine the cause and potential therapy; and to assess the extent of complications and institute supportive care.

Evaluation of volume status is critical in the setting of low urine output and rising BUN and Cr. Accumulated fluid balance is useful. Direct measurement of central venous pressure or pulmonary capillary occlusion pressure is recommended to assist in the determination of intravascular volume status and to optimize renal perfusion in the perioperative or post-injury patient.

Serum and urine chemistries can assist the clinician in the diagnosis and management of the patient with oliguria (Table 1.4). The fractional excretion of sodium (FENa) and urine sodium are useful measurements of how actively the kidney is resorbing sodium and reflect renal perfusion and intravascular volume status. In prerenal ARF, the kidney is hypoperfused; therefore, it actively resorbs Na and both the urine Na and FENa are *low*. In contrast, renal parenchymal damage results in loss of resorption of Na and the urine Na and FENa are *high*. The urine sediment is also useful in establishing a diagnosis. Muddy brown coarse granular casts in the urine sediment are the classic finding in ATN while

TABLE 1.4. Indices that distinguish prerenal ARF from ATN.

Measurement	Prerenal ARF	ATN
Specific gravity	>1.020	< or ~1.010
FENa	<0.1–1%	> 1% preferably >3%
Urine osmolality	>500	<350 or ~300
Urine sodium	<20	>40
Serum BUN/Cr	>20	<15 or 10–15
Microscopic sediment	Hyaline casts	Brown granular casts

FENa = fractional excretion of sodium (%) = 100 × (urine Na × serum Cr)/ (urine Cr × serum Na).
BUN/Cr = blood urea nitrogen-to-creatinine ratio.
CrCl = creatinine clearance = urine Cr × [timed urine volume (ml/min)]/ serum Cr.

white cell casts with eosinophiluria are seen in interstitial nephritis. Urine which dips positive for blood in the absence of red blood cells (RBCs/HPF) on microscopic examination suggests hemoglobinuria or myoglobinuria is present. This combination suggests that rhabdomyolysis or hemolysis as the cause of ARF.

Renal ultrasound imaging should be considered early to rule out obstruction in ARF. It documents that both kidneys are present and may identify other pathology while duplex scanning can demonstrate renal blood flow. Renal ultrasound also allows determination of kidney size with the finding of small kidneys indicating a chronic condition with superimposed acute deterioration.

Therapy

Therapeutic options for ARF depend on its cause. Prerenal ARF is diagnosed and treated by restoration of renal perfusion. Postrenal ARF frequently requires mechanical intervention, which may be as simple as placement of a Foley catheter or require abdominal decompression. *There is no known therapy to modify the course of Acute Tubular Necrosis (ATN) once established.* The clinician must strive to remove the cause of the disease and provide supportive care until the return of adequate renal function.

Restoration of intravascular volume. Even in patients that are clinically suspected of having ATN, intravascular volume should be normalized as assessed by clinical findings and the monitoring of arterial blood pressure and cardiac filling pressures (preload) utilizing either central venous pressure (>12 mmHg) or pulmonary capillary occlusion pressure(>15 mmHg). If the patient does not respond appropriately to volume loading with increased central venous pressure and increased urine output, a pulmonary artery catheter should be utilized to measure cardiac output and oxygen delivery. Even if hemodynamic parameters appear adequate a trial of fluid is recommended early in the course of oliguric ARF.

Diuretics. If renal function does not improve significantly after optimization of intravascular volume a trial of furosemide (40–320 mg IV in increasing doses) or mannitol (12.5–25 g IV) is recommended. These agents help convert oliguric ARF to non-oliguric ARF. If the urine output does not respond to the initial dose of mannitol, it should be stopped since the intravascular osmotic load can cause exacerbation of fluid overload and pulmonary or cerebral edema. If urine output does not respond to furosemide, then it should be combined with metolazone (5–10 mg orally) or chlorothiazide (500 mg IV). Care must be exercised in avoiding repeated doses of furosemide in the setting of anuria as complications including deafness and allergic interstitial nephritis are reported. In patients that respond to diuretics an individual agent or combination furosemide/mannitol drip can be used and titrated to response(a common recipe is 250 ml of D5W, 200 mg of furosemide, and 12.5 g of mannitol).

Vasopressors. Once intravascular volume has been restored, some patients remain hypotensive (mean arterial pressure <70). In these patients autoregulation of renal blood flow may be lost. Restoration of MAP to near normal levels is likely to increase GFR. In patients with chronic hypertension or renovascular disease a MAP of 75–80 mmHg may still be inadequate. No vasoactive agent has proven advantageous over another in the management of hypotension and oliguria. In patients with septic shock, profound hypotension, and oliguria, vasopressor therapy with norepinephrine may actually *improve* renal function by enhancing renal perfusion pressure to a greater extent than its vasoconstriction effects. The agent of choice likely will reflect the underlying pathophysiology (sepsis – norepinephrine; heart failure – dobutamine or milrinone).While a renal vasodilator dose of dopamine (1–3 μg/kg/min) may stimulate urine volume, it does not improve GFR, shorten the duration of ARF, or decrease the requirement for dialysis. In addition, dopamine may induce significant arrhythmias and possibly intestinal ischemia. Recent studies involving low-dose dopamine have been meta-analyzed and the results are that low-dose dopamine is not different from placebo in its effects on GFR.

Specific therapies. Patients with myoglobinuria require additional specific therapy: first, it is necessary to push urine output much higher than is necessary for fluid and electrolyte balance. Urine output should be maintained at >150 ml/h through the initial phases of treatment so as to dilute and clear precipitated and free myoglobin from the tubules. Although neither has been shown to be beneficial in controlled trials, it is recommended that the normovolemic patient with ongoing IV fluid resuscitation receive mannitol (1 g/kg initially) to further induce an osmotic diuresis and perhaps for an antioxidant effect. Second, urine pH should be increased above 7 since myoglobin precipitation is lower at alkaline pHs. This is accomplished by adding sodium bicarbonate to the IV fluids, monitoring urine pH at frequent intervals, and utilizing diuretics that promote an alkaline urine such as the carbonic anhydrase-inhibitor acetazolamide rather than furosemide, which tends to create an acidic urine. The overall goal is to produce a high-output *alkaline diuresis*.

In patients with acute abdominal compartment syndrome, therapy is directed at relieving the intraabdominal hypertension.

This is most readily accomplished by laparotomy. Standard medical therapy of ARF with volume loading and inotropes usually is ineffective in this setting; however, the response to abdominal decompression is usually dramatic and life-saving. The remaining wound is covered with an impermeable plastic drape to reduce fluid losses through the temporary abdominal wall hernia.

Complications

The mainstay of therapy for ARF is to control complications until return of adequate renal function (Table 1.5). Initial complications reflect the kidney's role as the primary regulator of volume and mineral balance. Subsequently, patients develop uremic symptoms, reflecting the importance of the kidney in excretion of nitrogenous waste.

In oliguric patients, fluid intake must be rigorously monitored. A reasonable goal is for input 1/4 output, or the volume of maintenance fluids to equal measured fluid losses (urine, gastrointestinal fluid, surgical drains) plus insensible losses, which can be estimated at 600 ml/day(higher if patient is febrile). Nutritional support in the setting of acute renal failure should have the same goals of caloric and nitrogen equilibrium as the surgical patient without ARF.

Potassium should almost never be administered to an oliguric patient. A particularly deceptive and dangerous situation is the patient with high-output ATN in which potentially large volumes of urine are produced but potassium is not excreted. Hyperkalemia can develop rapidly in this situation if normal urine losses are assumed and electrolyte replacement is performed empirically. Another worrisome situation for rapid development of hyperkalemia is clinical rhabdomyolysis. Here the muscle necrosis releases large amounts of potassium and phosphorus frequently resulting in the need for aggressive therapy and not infrequently, early dialysis. The first and immediate treatment for symptomatic hyperkalemia (K + >6.5 or significant EKG findings of peaked T-waves, widening of

TABLE 1.5. Complications of acute renal failure.

Complication	Clinical consequence	Therapy
Volume overload	Pulmonary edema	Fluid and sodium restriction
	Respiratory failure	Diuretics
Hyperkalemia	Arrhythmia	Potassium restriction
	Ventricular tachycardia	Calcium gluconate (10%)
	Heart block	Glucose (D50) and insulin
		Sodium bicarbonate (7.5%)
		Cation-exchange resin
Metabolic acidosis	Hyperventilation	Sodium bicarbonate for <15 meq/l
Hyponatremia	Water imbalance	Fluid restriction
Hypocalcemia	Carpopedal spasm	Phosphate binding antacids
Hyperphosphatemia	Arrhythmia	Avoid magnesium antacids
Hypermagnesemia		Supplemental calcium
Uremic syndrome	Nausea and vomiting	Renal replacement therapy
	Pericarditis or pleuritis	Hemodialysis
	Mental status changes	Hemofiltration
	Anemia	
	Platelet dysfunction	

QRS complex) is 10% Calcium Gluconate (5–10 ml IV over 2 min) which antagonizes the cardiac and neuromuscular effects. Glucose (50 ml of D50), Insulin (5–10 units regular IV over 5 min), and Sodium Bicarbonate (50 ml IV over 5 min) have an onset of 30–60 min and work primarily by shifting potassium into cells. Binding resins (15–30 g of resin in 50–100 ml of 20% sorbitol p.o. or by enema Q4 h) have an onset of several hours and exchange potassium for sodium.

Renal replacement. Several approaches to renal replacement therapy are available for the surgical patient in ARF. Intermittent hemodialysis has the greatest experience and established efficacy; however, over the last decade the availability of highly permeable membranes has allowed development of continuous renal replacement therapy (CRRT) which gradually removes fluids and solutes, resulting in better hemodynamic stability, and fluid and solute control (see Table 1.6). Dialysis therapy is indicated when the level of waste products in the blood is toxic or when fluid balance cannot be maintained with the use of medication or restriction. There is no evidence that dialysis shortens the course of ARF and because of potential complications of this therapy it should be reserved

TABLE 1.6. Comparison of continuous renal replacement therapy techniques (CRRT).

	SCUF	CAVH	CVVH	CAVHD	CVVHD
Access	A-V	A-V	V-V	A-V	V-V
Pump	No	No	Yes	No	Yes
Filtrate (ml/h)	100	600	1,000	300	300
Filtrate (l/day)	2.4	14.4	24	7.2	7.2
Dialysate flow (l/h)	0	0	0	1	1
Replacement fluid (l/day)	0	12	21.6	4.8	4.8
Urea clearance (ml/min)	1.7	10	16.7	21.7	21.7
Simplicity	1	2	3	2	3

Simplicity ranked 1–3: 1 = most simple, 3 = most difficult.
SCUF, slow continuous ultra-filtration; CAVH, continuous arterio-venous hemofiltration; CVVH, continuous veno-venous hemofiltration; CAVHD, continuous arterio-venous hemodialysis; CVVHD, continuous veno-venous hemodialysis.

for well documented complications of ARF. These are listed in Table 1.6 and include volume overload, acidosis, hyperkalemia, coma or seizure, uremic bleeding, and pericarditis. Absolute levels of BUN or Cr are not as important a factor in the decision to start dialysis as the patient's overall condition.

Regular dialysis 3 × weekly for 4 h at a blood flow rate of 200 ml/min gives the patient the equivalent of an average weekly glomerular filtration rate (GFR) of 10–15 ml/min. Unfortunately, intermittent hemodialysis in the ICU setting is frequently associated with hypotension, hypoxemia, and cardiac arrhythmias which limit the actual time for solute and fluid removal.

Patients that will not tolerate intermittent hemodialysis can be provided renal replacement through the use of a variety of continuous, lower flow techniques that differ in the access utilized and in the principal method of solute clearance. The simplest is slow continuous ultrafiltration (SCUF) which uses mean arterial pressure as the driving force. A dialysate solution can be added to the hemofiltration to assist solute removal. This is termed continuous arteriovenous hemodialysis (CAVHD). If mean arterial pressure is inadequate (MAP < 70–80), use of a pump within a veno-venous circuit can be utilized as an alternative. This is termed continuous veno-venous hemofiltration or hemodialysis (CVVH or CVVHD). The advantages of continuous techniques are that they are well tolerated in hypotension and allow a greater volume of fluid removal, facilitating nutritional support, compared to intermittent hemodialysis. Disadvantages of this approach are the need for anticoagulation and the high volume of replacement fluid that must be closely monitored.

Selected Readings

Bellomo R, Ronco C, Kellum J, et al., and the ADQI workgroup (2004) Acute renal failure – definition, outcome measures, animal models, fluid therapy and information technology needs: the Second International Consensus Conference of the ADQI Group. Crit Care 8: R204–212

Better O, Stein J (1990) Early management of shock and prophylaxis of acute renal failure in traumatic rhabdomyolysis. NEJM 322:825–829

Kellum J, Angus D, Johnson J, et al. (2002) Continuous versus intermittent renal replacement therapy: a meta-analysis. Intensive Care Med 28:29–37

McNelis J, Marini C, Simms H (2003) Abdominal compartment syndrome: clinical manifestations and predictive factors. Curr Opin Crit Care 9:133–136

Meschi M, Detrenis S, Musini S, et al. (2006) Facts and fallacies concerning the prevention of contrast medium-induced nephropathy. Crit Care Med 34:2060–2068

Mindell J, Chertow G (1997) A practical approach to acute renal failure. Med Clin North Am 81:731–748

Schenarts P, Sagraves S, Bard M, et al. (2006) Low-dose dopa-mine: a physiologically based review. Curr Surg 63:219–225

Swan S (1997) Aminoglycoside nephrotoxicity. Semin Nephrol 17:27–33

2
Monitoring of Respiratory Function and Weaning from Mechanical Ventilation

Philip S. Barie and Soumitra R. Eachempati

Pearls and Pitfalls

- The most common reason for mechanical ventilation is to decrease the work of breathing, but other goals include improved gas exchange, resting of respiratory muscles, and prevention of deconditioning.
- Modes of mechanical, machine-delivered breaths triggered by the patient's own inspiratory efforts are preferred.
- Oxygen toxicity should be minimized by using a F_IO_2 which keeps arterial oxygen tension $(PaO_2) > 60$ mmHg or oxygen saturation $> 88\%$.
- Ideal tidal volumes are about 6 ml/kg and plateau airway pressures should be <35 cm H_2O.
- Use of 5 cm PEEP restores functional residual capacity.
- Although most conscious patients require some form of sedation during mechanical ventilation, sedation should be minimized with daily sedation "holidays" of spontaneous breathing.
- The concept of a "ventilator bundle" optimizes mechanical ventilation and includes 30 degree elevation of the head of the bed, prophylaxis against deep vein thrombosis and gastric stress ulceration, and daily sedation holiday.
- Pulse oximetry measures oxygen saturation very accurately above 70% but requires pulsatile flow; hypothermia, hypotension, peripheral vascular disease, and the use of

K.I. Bland et al. (eds.), *Critical Care Surgery*,
DOI 10.1007/978-1-84996-378-7_2,
© Springer-Verlag London Limited 2011

vasoconstrictor medications will interfere with readings from a pulse oximeter.

- Several newer non-invasive methods of monitoring cardiac output include thoracic bioimpedance, esophageal Doppler measurements, and near-infrared spectroscopy; these techniques are not available universally and have their own disadvantages and disadvantages.
- For arterial monitoring of blood gases or blood pressure, the brachial artery and the femoral artery should be avoided whenever possible.
- Pulmonary artery catheters are used to measure cardiac output, mixed venous oxygen saturation, and preload; the latter is estimated from the wedge pressure which approximates left atrial pressure, in indication of left ventricular end-diastolic pressure.
- Methods of weaning include the trial of spontaneous breathing, combination of SIMV (synchronized intermittent mechanical ventilation), and pressure support. Measurements of maximal negative inspiratory pressure, vital capacity, and minute volume help identify appropriate candidates.
- When weaning a patient from mechanical ventilation, intolerance is evident by increase in respiratory rate, decrease in tidal volume, and increased work of breathing (oxygen requirements), which can lead to decreased oxygen delivery, CO_2 retention, and increased cardiac stress.

Increasing patient acuity requires sophisticated methods to monitor and support these critically ill patients. Mechanical ventilation, a mainstay of modern ICU care, may be required to manage airway patency and support acute respiratory failure. New technology provides several modes of ventilation, with the goals of improved gas exchange, better patient comfort, and ultimately, rapid liberation from the ventilator. During acute respiratory failure, the work of breathing necessary to initiate a breath increases four-to six-fold. The most common reason to initiate mechanical ventilation is to decrease the patient's work of breathing. Additional goals include improved gas exchange, enhanced coordination between support and the patients' own efforts, resting of respiratory muscles, prevention of de-conditioning, and prevention of iatrogenic, ventilator-induced lung injury while promoting healing.

Nearly all ventilators can be set to allow full patient support or periods of exercise (i.e., periods promoting the work of breathing). Thus, choice of ventilator settings is often a matter of physician preference, modifying how positive airway pressure is applied and the interplay between mechanical support and the patients' own efforts. Unless appropriate settings are chosen to synchronize with the patient's own efforts, mechanical ventilation can cause increased work of breathing. Complete suppression of spontaneous breathing leads rapidly to respiratory muscle atrophy, therefore modes of mechanical ventilation are preferred wherein machine-delivered breaths are triggered by the patients' own inspiratory efforts, so as to maintain readiness for the patient to resume the work of breathing once the acute episode resolves, facilitating weaning and liberation from the ventilator.

Routine Ventilator Settings

Ventilator settings are based on the patient's ideal body mass and medical condition, manipulating, at minimum, respiratory rate, tidal volume (V_T), and fraction of inspired oxygen (F_IO_2). The risk of oxygen toxicity is minimized by using the lowest F_IO_2 that can oxygenate arterial blood satisfactorily to maintain arterial oxygen tension (PaO_2)>60 mmHg or oxygen saturation (SaO_2) >88%.

Although normal lungs may be ventilated safely with V_T 8–10 ml/kg for prolonged periods, convincing data indicate that a lesser V_T (6 ml/kg) prevents alveolar overdistention in acute lung injury and acute respiratory distress syndrome (ARDS); a lesser V_T helps to decrease endothelial, epithelial, and basement membrane injuries associated with ventilator-induced lung injury. Plateau airway pressure (P_{plat}), measured in a relaxed patient by occluding the ventilator circuit briefly at end-inspiration, should be kept ≤ 35 cm H_2O. Low V_T ventilation may lead to an increase in $PaCO_2$. Acceptance of an increased $PaCO_2$ in exchange for controlled alveolar pressure is termed *permissive hypercapnia*. It is important to focus on pH rather than $PaCO_2$ during permissive hypercapnia. If the pH decreases to <7.25, respirator rates should be increased or $NaHCO_3$ can be administered.

The respirator rate set on the ventilator depends on the mode. With conventional, assist-control ventilation (ACV), the backup rate should be about four breaths/min less than the patient's spontaneous rate to ensure that the ventilator will continue to supply adequate minute ventilation should the patient have a sudden decrease in spontaneous breathing. With synchronized, intermittent mandatory ventilation (SIMV), the respiratory rate is typically set high at first and then decreased gradually in accordance with patient tolerance.

An inspiratory gas flow rate of 60 l/min is used with most patients during ACV and SIMV. If the flow rate is insufficient to meet the patient's requirements, the patient will strain against his/her own pulmonary impedance and that of the ventilator, with a consequent increase in work of breathing (and thus oxygen/energy consumption).

In the ACV and SIMV modes, the patient must lower airway pressure below a preset threshold (usually minus 1–2 cm H_2O) in order to trigger the ventilator to deliver a tidal breath. Pressure support is an accepted method of assisting spontaneous breathing in a ventilated patient, either partially or fully. The patient triggers the ventilator, which delivers a flow of gas in response up to a preset pressure limit(e.g., 10 cm H_2O) depending on the desired minute ventilation. The gas flow then cycles off when a certain percentage of peak inspiratory flow (usually 25%) is reached. Tidal volumes may vary, just as they do spontaneously.

Positive end-expiratory pressure (PEEP), also referred to as continuous positive airway pressure (CPAP), is added to restore functional residual capacity (FRC) to normal for the patient (usually 5 cm H_2O, absent acute respiratory failure requiring higher therapeutic PEEP).When lung volumes are low, the work of breathing during early inhalation is decreased. Non-compliant lungs require higher intrapleural pressures to inflate to a normal tidal volume, even with CPAP. Addition of pressure support assists the patient to move up the pressure-volume curve (larger changes in volume for a given applied pressure for patients with increased lung compliance).Pressure support ventilation describes the combination of pressure support and PEEP (or CPAP). Although useful in the patient breathing spontaneously, pressure support may also be used to assist spontaneous breaths in SIMV. Weaning maybe facilitated using this combination, as the backup (SIMV)rate is weaned initially, and then the pressure support.

Sedation

Most patients who require mechanical ventilation will require sedation, but only a minority (~10%) will also require neuromuscular blockade. Multiple pharmacologic agents are available for sedation (Table 2.1), so the choice of agent can be individualized for the patient, but caution must be used to assure that patients are not over-sedated. Titration of sedation to patient comfort is facilitated by providing sedation titrated to a sedation score of 3–4 points on the Ramsay or Riker scale (Table 2.2). Intermittent doses of sedatives are often preferred to continuous infusions in an attempt to minimize the amount of sedation. Neuromuscular blockade should be avoided whenever possible because of patient discomfort, worry of ventilator failure or disconnection, and muscular deconditioning.

Prolonged or excessive sedation increases the duration of mechanical ventilation and increases the likelihood of ventilator-associated pneumonia and the need for tracheostomy. Protocolized weaning of sedative medications and daily sedation "holidays" to permit trials of spontaneous breathing help to lessen the duration of mechanical ventilation and decrease the risk of pneumonia and other complications.

TABLE 2.1. Selected formulary for analgesia, anesthesia, and sedation in the ICU.

Agent	Initial IV adult dose
Induction agents	
Etomidate	6 mg or more
Ketamine	1–2 mg/kg
Propofol	1.5–2.5 mg/kg
Intravenous sedatives/analgesics	
Midazolam	0.5–4 mg
Lorazepam	1–4 mg
Morphine	2–10 mg
Hydromorphone	0.5–2.0 mg
Fentanyl	50–100 mcg
Neuromuscular blocking agents	
Succinylcholine	0.75–1.5 mg/kg
Atracurium	0.2–0.5 mg/kg
Cisatracurium	0.2–0.5 mg/kg
Pancuronium	0.05–0.1 mg
Vecuronium	0.08–0.10 mg/kg
Miscellaneous agents	
Dexmedetomidine	1 mcg/kg load, then 0.2–0.7 mcg/kg/h
Haloperidol	2–5 mg
Ketorolac	0.5–1.0 mg/kg
Reversal agents	
Flumazenil	0.1–0.2 mg
Naloxone	up to 0.4 mg
Edrophonium *with*	0.5–1.0 mg/kg
Atropine	0.007–0.014 mg/kg
Neostigmine *with*	0.5–2.0 mg
Glycopyrrolate	0.1–0.2 mg

Dosages should be adjusted as appropriate for renal or hepatic insufficiency.

TABLE 2.2. Sedation scales in common usage.

	Value	Clinical correlate
Ramsey sedation score		
Awake scores 1–3	1	Anxious, agitated, or restless
	2	Cooperative, oriented, tranquil
	3	Responsive to commands
Asleep scores 4–6	4	Brisk response to stimulus[a]
	5	Sluggish response to stimulus
	6	No response to stimulus
Riker sedation-agitation scale		
Dangerous agitation	7	Pulling at catheters, striking staff
Very agitated	6	Does not calm to voice, requires restraint
Agitated	5	Anxious, responds to verbal cues
Calm and cooperative	4	Calm, awakens easily, follows commands
Sedated	3	Awakens to stimulus
Very sedated	2	Arouses to stimulus, does not follow commands
Unarousable	1	Minimal or no response to noxious stimulus

[a]Stimulus: light glabellar tap or loud auditory stimulus.

Ventilator Bundle

Care of the patient on mechanical ventilation is more than just providing ventilation and oxygenation. Such patients are at risk for numerous complications, not all of which are related directly to acute respiratory failure or the actual mechanical ventilation. The clinician must bear in mind the total patient. Prolonged bed rest increases deconditioning, venous thromboembolic complications, and development of pressure ulcers. Neurologic compromise from disease or sedative/analgesic drugs may impair the sensorium, increasing the risk of pulmonary aspiration of gastric contents. Oversedation may contribute directly to the need for prolonged mechanical ventilation, which is a definite risk factor for ventilator-associated pneumonia (incidence ~2%/day of ventilation). Prolonged ventilation (>48 h) also increases the risk of stress-related gastric mucosal hemorrhage.

Several "best practices" have been combined into a ventilator bundle to optimize the outcomes of mechanical ventilation, including four maneuvers: keeping the head of the bed up at least 30 degrees from level at all times unless contraindicated medically, prophylaxis against venous thromboembolic disease, prophylaxis against stress-related gastric mucosal hemorrhage, and a daily "sedation holiday" to assess for readiness to liberate from mechanical ventilation through assessment by a trial of spontaneous breathing. Careful adoption and adherence to all facets of this "ventilator bundle" can decrease the risk of pneumonia along with other maneuvers, such as adherence to the principles of infection control.

Monitoring of Mechanical Ventilation

Blood Gas Monitoring

Blood gas analyzers measure blood pO_2, pCO_2, and pH. Hemoglobin saturation is calculated from pO_2 using the oxyhemoglobin dissociation curve, assuming a normal P50 (the pO_2 at which SaO_2 is 50%, normally 26.6 mmHg), and normal hemoglobin structure. Blood gas analyzers with a co-oximeter measure the various forms of hemoglobin directly, including oxyhemoglobin, total hemoglobin, carboxyhemoglobin, and methemoglobin. The bicarbonate, standard bicarbonate, and base excess, however, are calculated from the pH and pCO_2.

A fresh, heparinized, bubble-free arterial blood sample is required. Heparin is acidic; if present in excess, pCO_2 and HCO_3 are decreased spuriously. Delay in obtaining these measurements from an arterial blood sample allows continued metabolism by erythrocytes which decrease the pH and pO_2 and increase the pCO_2. An iced specimen can be assayed accurately for up to 1h. Air bubbles decrease pCO_2 and increase pO_2.

The solubility of all gases in blood increases with a decrease in temperature, thus hypothermia causes pO_2 and pCO_2 to decrease and pH to increase. Analysis at 37°C of a sample taken from a hypothermic patient will cause a somewhat spurious increase in pO_2 and pCO_2, but the error is usually not meaningful.

Non-invasive Monitoring

Pulse oximetry: Pulse oximetry detects even slight decreases in SaO_2 with only about a 60-s delay. The device calculates SaO_2 by estimating the difference in signal intensity between oxygenated and deoxygenated blood from red (660 nm) and near-infrared (940 nm) light. Pulse oximetry requires pulsatile blood flow to be accurate (Table 2.3), but all things being equal, data can be obtained from a detector on the finger, earlobe, or forehead. Pulse oximetry is very accurate (2%) for SaO_2 from 70% to 100%, but less so below 70%.

Several aspects of the technology and patient physiology limit the accuracy of pulse oximetry. If the device cannot detect pulsatile flow, the waveform will be dampened. Consequently, pulse oximetry may be inaccurate in patients with hypothermia, hypotension, hypovolemia, or peripheral vascular disease, or in patients being treated with vasoconstrictor medications. Additionally, an increased carboxy hemoglobin concentration will lead to a falsely increased SaO_2, because its reflected light is absorbed at the same wavelength as oxyhemoglobin. Other causes of inaccurate pulse oximetry include ambient light and motion artifact.

TABLE 2.3. Sources of error in pulse oximetry.

False depression of SaO_2
Methemoglobinemia (reads at 85%)
Methylene blue dye
Indocyanine green dye
Non-pulsatile blood flow (no reading may be appreciable at all)
Vasoconstriction
Hypotension
Hypothermia
Hypovolemia
Venous congestion with exaggerated venous pulsation
Peripheral edema
Nail polish
Fluorescent lighting
Use of electrocautery (electrical interference)
Severe anemia (Hemoglobin concentration 3–4 g/dl)
Shivering (may cause mechanical loss of signal)
False elevation of SaO_2
Carboxyhemoglobin
No effect
Fatal hemoglobin
Hyperbilirubinemia

Capnography: Capnography measures the concentration of CO_2 in expired gas. This technique is most reliable in ventilated patients and employs either mass spectroscopy or infrared light absorption to detect CO_2. The peak CO_2 concentration occurs at end-exhalation and is regarded as the patient's "end-tidal CO_2" ($ETCO_2$), which approximates the alveolar gas concentration (Fig. 2.1). Capnography is useful to assess the success of airway intubation, weaning from mechanical

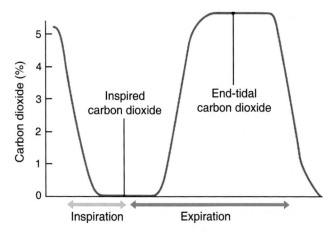

FIGURE 2.1. A normal capnograph tracing.

ventilation, and resuscitation (Table 2.4). Detection of hypercarbia during ventilator weaning can diminish the need for blood gas determinations. Used with pulse oximetry, many patients can be liberated from mechanical ventilation without reliance on blood gases or invasive monitoring.

The characteristics of the waveform provides information about the patient's pulmonary status and in particular whether obstructive disease or inadequate ventilation is present. A sudden decrease or even disappearance of $ETCO_2$ can be correlated with potentially serious pathology or events, such as a low cardiac output state, disconnection from the ventilator, or pulmonary thromboembolism (Table 2.5). A gradual increase of $ETCO_2$ can be seen with hypoventilation; the converse is also true. Another cause of a gradually decreasing $ETCO_2$ is hypovolemia.

Non-invasive Cardiac Output

Thoracic bioimpedance: Thoracic bioimpedance determines cardiac output by deriving information from topical electrodes placed on the anterior chest and neck, estimating the

TABLE 2.4. Changes in end-tidal CO_2 ($ETCO_2$).

Increased $ETCO_2$
  Decreased alveolar ventilation
    Reduced respiratory rate
  Reduced tidal volume
  Increased equipment dead space
Increased CO_2 production
  Fever
  Hypercatabolic state
  Excess feeding with carbohydrate
Increased inspired CO_2 concentration
  CO_2 absorber exhausted
  Increased CO_2 in inspired gas
  Rebreathing of expired gas
Decreased $ETCO_2$
  Increased alveolar ventilation
    Increased respiratory rate
    Increased tidal volume
Decreased CO_2 production
  Hypothermia
  Hypocatabolic state
Increased alveolar dead space
  Decreased cardiac output
  Pulmonary embolism (clot, air, fat)
  High positive end-expiratory pressure (PEEP)
Sampling error
  Air in sample line (no or diminished signal)
  Water in sample line (no or diminished signal)
  Inadequate tidal volume (no or diminished signal)
  Disconnection of monitor from tubing (no signal)
  Artificial airway not in trachea (e.g., esophageal intubation) (no signal)

TABLE 2.5. Indications and contraindications for central venous pressure monitoring and pulmonary artery catheterization.

Central venous pressure monitoring

Indications

Major operative procedures involving large fluid shifts or blood loss

Hypovolemia or shock

Intravascular volume assessment when urine output is not reliable or unavailable (e.g., renal failure)

Major trauma

Surgical procedures with a high risk of air embolism, such as sitting-position craniotomy or major liver resection

Frequent venous blood sampling

Venous access for vasoactive or irritating drugs

Chronic drug administration

Inadequate peripheral IV access

Rapid infusion of IV fluids (using large cannulae)

Parenteral nutrition

Insertion of other devices

PA catheters

Transvenous pacing wires

Access for renal replacement therapy

Contraindications

Absolute

Infection at the site of insertion

Large tricuspid valve vegetations

Superior vena cava syndrome

Tumor or thrombus in the right atrium

Relative

(continued)

TABLE 2.5. (continued)

Anticoagulant therapy

Coagulopathy

Contralateral diaphragm dysfunction (risk of recurrent nerve injury with internal jugular cannulation)

Newly inserted pacemaker wires

Presence of carotid disease

Recent cannulation of the internal jugular vein

Thyromegaly or prior neck surgery (especially ipsilateral carotid endarterectomy)

Pulmonary artery catheterization

Indications

Cardiac surgery

Poor left ventricular function (ejection fraction <0.4; end-diastolic pressure >18 mmHg)

Recent myocardial infarction

Complications of myocardial infarction (e.g., mitral insufficiency, ventricular septal defect, ventricular aneurysm)

Combined lesions, e.g., coronary artery disease with mitral insufficiency or aortic stenosis

Asymmetric septal hypertrophy

Intraaortic balloon pump

Non-cardiac indications

Shock of any cause

Severe pulmonary disease

Complicated surgical procedures

Multiple trauma

Hepatic transplantation

Aortic surgery

Contraindications

(continued)

TABLE 2.5.   (continued)

The same contraindications for central venous catheterization apply here. Additionally

Absolute

Tricuspid or pulmonary valvular stenosis

Right ventricular masses (tumor or thrombus)

Tetralogy of Fallot

Relative

Ventricular arrhythmia

left ventricular systolic time interval from time 1/m-derivative bioimpedance signals. The lag time for the system to provide data is approximately 2–5 min from initial lead placement and activation. The main drawback of thoracic bioimpedance is that it is susceptible to any alteration of the electrode contact or positioning on the patient.

Esophageal Doppler: The esophageal Doppler monitor (EDM) device is a soft, 6 mm catheter placed noninvasively into the esophagus. A Doppler flow probe at its tip allows continuous monitoring of cardiac output and stroke volume. A 4-MHz continuous wave ultrasound frequency is reflected to produce a waveform, representing the change in blood flow in the descending aorta (about 80% of cardiac output) with each pulsation. EDM maybe more accurate than a pulmonary artery catheter (see below) in patients with cardiac valvular lesions, septal defects, arrhythmias, or pulmonary hypertension. The primary disadvantage of EDM is loss of waveform with only slight positional changes, leading to dampened, inaccurate readings.

Near-infrared spectroscopy: Near-infrared spectroscopy measures tissue O_2 tension non-invasively in close to real time. Near-infrared light of four calibrated wavelengths penetrates tissue to a depth of approximately 15 mm below the sensor, which is placed usually on the thenar eminence. Analysis of reflected light produces an absolute measurement of tissue oxygenation (StO_2) in the skeletal muscle microcirculation, which has been evaluated in a wide range of experimental conditions. Skeletal muscle StO_2 has been found to correlatewithO_2 delivery, base deficit, and serum lactate concentration in experimental and clinical hemorrhagic shock. Detection is possible over a StO_2 range of 1–99% but is most accurate for $StO_2 > 70\%$.

In a recent multicenter trial of 383 patients with major trauma who required blood transfusion, 50 of whom eventually developed multiple organ dysfunction syndrome, the monitoring with near-infrared spectroscopy was begun within 30 min of arrival in the emergency department and continued for 24 h. A $StO_2 > 75\%$ maintained during the first hour of monitoring indicated adequate tissue perfusion with affected patients having an 88% survival. In contrast, an $StO_2 < 75\%$ in the first hour was predictive of development of multiple organ dysfunction syndrome (78%); 91% of those patients died.

Invasive Hemodynamic Monitoring

Arterial catheterization: Measurement of arterial blood pressure is the most reproducible method of evaluating hemodynamics. For stable patients, automated non-invasive blood pressure cuff devices can measure blood pressure accurately and precisely (error, ±2%), as often as every 5 min. Blood pressure will be overestimated if the cuff is too small and if systolic blood pressure is less than 60 mmHg. Arrhythmias such as atrial fibrillation degrade accuracy. If blood pressure fluctuates more frequently than intermittent measurements can capture, continuous monitoring is needed via an indwelling arterial catheter.

Indications for invasive arterial monitoring include prolonged operations (>4 h in duration), unstable hemodynamics, substantial blood loss, frequent blood sampling, or a need for precise control of blood pressure (e.g., neurosurgical patients and patients on cardiopulmonary bypass). Patients on mechanical ventilation or inotropic support often benefit from arterial catheterization. Although there is morbidity from the insertion and the indwelling catheter, there is also morbidity from repetitive arterial punctures; the risk: benefit analysis is a matter of clinical judgment for "less unstable" patients.

Arterial catheters may be placed in any of several locations. The radial artery at the wrist is used most commonly; the ulnar artery is usually larger but is relatively inaccessible to percutaneous access. To minimize the possibility of hand ischemia from arterial occlusion or embolization of debris or clot from the catheter tip, careful confirmation of the patency of the collateral circulation of the hand is mandatory before arterial cannulation at the wrist. Alternative sites include the umbilical artery (in neonates) and the axillary and superficial femoral arteries in adults; the latter is not a location of choice because the burden of plaque (and therefore risk of distal embolization) is higher, as is the infection rate. The brachial artery should be avoided; the collateral circulation around the elbow is poor, and the risk of ischemia of the hand or forearm is too great.

Because the arterial waveform may be damped by severe peripheral vasoconstriction during vasopressor therapy, it may be necessary to use a longer catheter at a more central location (e.g., axillary, femoral) to position the catheter tip into an unaffected artery in the torso. Nosocomial infection of arterial catheters is unusual provided basic tenets of infection control are honored, and femoral artery catheterization is avoided. Other complications from arterial catheterization include bleeding, hematoma, and pseudoaneurysm formation.

Central venous pressure monitoring: The central venous pressure (CVP) is an interplay of the circulating blood volume, venous tone, and right ventricular function. By measuring the filling pressure of the right ventricle, the CVP provides an estimate of the status of the intravascular volume. Indications for cannulation of a central vein are numerous, and the contraindications are relatively few (Table 2.5). Strict adherence to asepsis, full barrier precautions, and adherence to the principles of infection control are crucial to avoid the potentially life-threatening complication of catheter-related blood stream infection. Central venous access can be obtained at several body sites, including the basilic, femoral, external jugular, internal jugular, or subclavian vein. The internal jugular, subclavian, and femoral veins are used most often, listed in decreasing frequency. The internal jugular vein is most popular site because of ease of accessibility, a high technical success rate, and a low complication rate, although the infection rate is higher than for subclavian vein catheters, allegedly because of more movement at the insertion site. The subclavian site is the most technically demanding for placement and has the highest rate of pneumothorax (1.5–3%), but the infection rate is the lowest of the three. The femoral vein site is least preferred, despite the relative ease of catheter placement. The femoral site is particularly prone to infection, and the risks of arterial puncture (9–15%) and venous thromboembolic complications are much higher than for jugular or subclavian venipuncture. Overall complications are comparable for internal jugular and subclavian vein cannulation (6–12%), and higher for femoral vein cannulation (13–19%).

Pulmonary artery catheterization: A pulmonary artery (Swan Ganz) catheter is a balloon-tipped, flow-directed catheter that is usually inserted percutaneously via a central vein; the balloon tip is then "floated" through the right side of the heart and into the pulmonary artery. This catheter typically contains several ports for pressure monitoring or fluid administration. Some pulmonary artery catheters include a sensor to measure central(mixed) venous oxygen saturation or right ventricular volume. Data from these catheters are used mainly to determine cardiac output and preload, which is stimulated most commonly by the pulmonary artery occlusion pressure (PAOP), so-called wedge pressure.

Normally, PAOP approximates left atrial pressure, which in turn approximates left ventricular end-diastolic pressure, itself a reflection of left ventricular end-diastolic volume, which represents preload, the actual target parameter. Many factors cause PAOP to reflect inaccurately the left ventricular end diastolic volume, including mitral stenosis, high levels of PEEP (>10 cm H_2O), and changes in left ventricular compliance (e.g., due to myocardial infarction, pericardial effusion, or increased afterload). Inaccurate readings may result from balloon overinflation, improper catheter position, alveolar pressure exceeding pulmonary venous pressure (as with high pressures of PEEP ventilation), or severe pulmonary hypertension. Increased PAOP occurs in left-sided heart failure, whereas decreased PAOP occurs with hypovolemia or decreased preload.

A desirable feature of pulmonary artery catheterization is the ability to measure central mixed venous oxygen saturation, although sampling from the superior vena cava via a CVP catheter may be comparable. Some catheters have embedded fiberoptic sensors that measure oxygen saturation directly. Causes of low central mixed venous oxygen saturation include anemia, pulmonary disease, carboxyhemoglobinemia, low cardiac output, and increased tissue oxygen demand. Ideally, the pulmonary mixed venous oxygen tension should be 35–40 mmHg, with a central mixed venous oxygen saturation of about 70%. Values of pulmonary mixed venous oxygen tension <30 mmHg are critically low.

No studies have demonstrated unequivocally that use of pulmonary artery catheters decreases morbidity or mortality; some retrospective data even suggest that they are associated with excess mortality. Critically ill patients who require one or more inotropic agents, despite resuscitation with large volumes of fluid, may benefit from such monitoring, both in the operating room and the ICU, but lack of demonstrable benefit has decreased the use of pulmonary artery catheters substantially.

Newer pulmonary artery catheters allow continuous monitoring of cardiac output and central mixed venous oxygen saturation. Continuous data may be useful when O_2 transport is marginal, such as patients with ARDS on high levels of PEEP. A recent large multicenter trial, however, conducted by the ARDSnet investigators, showed no benefit of pulmonary artery monitoring versus CVP monitoring of fluid administration for patients with ARDS. Complications of pulmonary arterial catheterizations include infection (2–5%), hemo-or pneumothorax (2–5%), migration (5–10%), patient discomfort, arrhythmia (10–15%), and hemorrhage (0.2%).

Rare complications include catheter knotting in the right ventricle (especially in patients with heart failure, cardiomyopathy, or pulmonary hypertension), pulmonary infarction, pulmonary artery or cardiac perforation, valvular injury, and endocarditis. Pulmonary artery rupture occurs in fewer than 0.1% of patients with pulmonary artery catheters and is generally fatal. Distal migration of the PAC within the pulmonary artery increases the risk dramatically of pulmonary artery rupture and is one of the few indications for routine daily bedside chest radiography for all patients with acute respiratory failure.

Liberation from Mechanical Ventilation

Objective measures and proactive strategies can hasten the liberation of patients from the ventilator. The stakes are high; each day of mechanical ventilation (e.g., endotracheal or tracheostomy tube) increases the need for sedation, which may postpone "liberation day." Moreover, each day of mechanical ventilation increases the risk of ventilator-associated pneumonia.

Failure to separate from the ventilator may be due to disease-or therapy-related reasons. Most clinical cases of failed liberation from the ventilator are multifactorial, but respiratory muscle fatigue is a common factor, in that the load on the respiratory system exceeds the capacity to breathe (Table 2.6). The increased load may take the form of a demand for increased minute ventilation or increased work of breathing. Increased minute ventilation may result from increased CO_2 production, increased dead space ventilation, or increased ventilatory drive. Increased CO_2 production may be caused by a catabolic state or overfeeding with carbohydrate. Increased dead space (ventilation of un- or under-perfused lung) may be caused by decreased cardiac output, pulmonary embolism, pulmonary hypertension, severe acute lung injury, or iatrogenically from ventilator-associated lung injury. Increased ventilatory drive may occur from muscle fatigue or failure, stimulation of pulmonary J receptors (usually by lung

TABLE 2.6. Load on the respiratory system.

Demand for increased minute ventilation
Increased carbon dioxide production
Increased dead space ventilation
Increased ventilatory drive
Increased work of breathing
Airway obstruction
Decreased respiratory system compliance
Decreased respiratory system capacity
Impaired central drive to breathe
Integrity of phrenic nerve transmission
Impaired respiratory muscle force generation

inflammation or parenchymal hemorrhage), or lesions of the central nervous system. Psychologic stress is also an important factor that may manifest itself as tachypnea, hypoxemia, agitation, or delirium. Stress may be caused by inadequate analgesia, sedation, or untreated delirium. Acute alcohol or drug withdrawal is a major factor in some patients.

Increased work of breathing results from either increased airflow resistance or decreased thoracic compliance. Airway obstruction can result from reversible small airways disease (e.g., bronchospasm), tracheal stenosis, tracheomalacia, glottic edema or dysfunction, mucus plugging, or muscle weakness. Muscle dysfunction may be caused by nutritional or metabolic causes (including hypocalcemia, hypokalemia, or hypophosphatemia). The critical illness polyneuropathy syndrome has a poorly understood pathophysiology but is associated with sepsis and often diagnosed when sought specifically by electromyography. Other potential causes of muscular failure or weakness include hypoxemia, hypercarbia, and possibly anemia.

Patients who "fight" the ventilator technically have the syndrome of patient-ventilator dyssynchrony. The cause must be sought; sedating the patient more deeply (or administering neuromuscular blockade) before a correctable cause is identified and remedied may be catastrophic if an unstable airway is the cause. A systematic approach to evaluation is advocated. Recognizing that patient and ventilator are supposed to be working in concert facilitates understanding that the problem maybe the patient or the ventilator. The cause may be found anywhere on the continuum from the alveolus to the power outlet or the source of respiratory gases (Table 2.7). The first step is always to ensure that the patient has a properly positioned, patent airway.

Liberation from mechanical ventilation may be easy to accomplish after short-term support. As many as 25% of all ventilated patients will experience respiratory distress during the initial weaning attempt, such that mechanical ventilation has to be reinstituted; patients recovering from acute respiratory failure, pneumonia, or major torso trauma can be especially challenging. Patients who cannot be weaned have a characteristic response to spontaneous breathing trials, including an almost-immediate increase in respiratory rate and decrease in tidal volume. As the trial continues over 30–60min, work of breathing increases substantially by four-to-sevenfold. Increased O_2 demand is met by increased O_2 extraction, which eventually causes decreased O_2 delivery and hypoxemia. Pulmonary compliance decreases, and the rapid, shallow breathing pattern causes CO_2 retention. There is considerable cardiovascular stress also, with increased afterload on both ventricles from the large changes in intrathoracic pressure generated by the struggling patient.

Timing is important; if weaning is delayed unnecessarily, the patient remains at risk for a host of ventilator-associated complications. If premature, weaning failure may lead to cardiopulmonary decompensation and need for prolonged ventilation. In general, discontinuation of mechanical ventilation is not attempted with unstable hemodynamics or if $PaO_2 < 60$ mmHg with $F_IO_2 \geq 0.60$.

Of note, adequate oxygenation alone does not predict successful weaning; more important is the ability of respiratory muscles to perform increased work. Decisions based solely on clinical judgment are frequently in error. Parameters gathered traditionally, including the maximal negative inspiratory

TABLE 2.7. Therapies to reverse ventilatory failure.

Improve muscular function

   Treat sepsis-avoid aminoglycosides

   Nutritional support without overfeeding (follow indirect calorimetry)

   Replete electrolytes to normal

   Assure periods of rest-do not exhaust the patient

   Limit neuromuscular blockade

   Avoid oversedation

   Identify/correct hypothyroidism

Reduce respiratory load

   Airway resistance

     Ensure airway patency/adequate caliber

   Compliance (elastance)

     Treat pneumonia

     Treat pulmonary edema

     Identify/reduce intrinsic PEEP (auto-PEEP)

     Drain large pleural effusions

     Evacuate pneumothorax

     Treat ileus (promotility agents)

     Decompress abdominal distention/treat abdominal compartment syndrome

     Position patient 30. head-up

   Minute ventilation

     Treat sepsis

     Antipyresis (T > 40°C?)

     Avoid overfeeding

     Correct metabolic acidosis

     Identify/reduce intrinsic PEEP (auto-PEEP)

   Bronchodilators

   Maintain least possible PEEP

   Resuscitate shock/correct hypovolemia

   Identify and treat pulmonary embolism

pressure, the vital capacity, and the minute volume, have limited predictive accuracy. Respiratory frequency (f)/V_T during 1 min of spontaneous breathing (the Rapid Shallow Breathing Index) is more accurate (95% probability of success) if f/V_T < 80 after a 30-min trial of spontaneous breathing.

The process of weaning begins by determining patient readiness (Table 2.8). Patients should be screened carefully for hemodynamic stability, cooperative mental status, respiratory muscle strength, consistent and adequate wakefulness, ability

TABLE 2.8. Cornell protocol for liberation from mechanical ventilation.

Screening (performed at least once daily, usually in early AM, by respiratory therapist, nurse, or physician, according to local protocol)

Resolution of the underlying disease process

No vasopressors or sedative infusions (except propofol or dexmedetomidine). No neuromuscular blocking agents

Intermittent doses of sedatives are permissible

No active myocardial ischemia or cardiac rhythm disturbances

V_E < 15 l/min

P_aO_2:F_IO_2 > 120 on F_IO_2 < 0.55

P_aCO_2 < 50 mmHg

Physiologic pH (7.30–7.50)

PEEP < 8 cm H_2O

Pressure support < 8 cm H_2O

Adequate cough/clearance of secretions

↓

YES = NO → Return to screening

↓

Proceed with spontaneous breathing trial-turn off enteral feedings and monitor serum glucose concentration closely, especially if on continuous infusion of insulin

(continued)

TABLE 2.8. (continued)

Spontaneous breathing trial

Calculate RSBI; target <105

↓

YES = NO → Return to screening — treat to reduce respiratory load

↓

Continue spontaneous breathing trial

CPAP with flow-by trigger, no change in CPAP or FIO2 over course of 1-h trial

Failure criteria

RR > 35 breaths/min for 5 min

SaO_2 < 90% for 30 s or more

HR > 140 beats/min, or sustained D > 20% in either direction

BP_{syst} > 180 mmHg or < 90 mmHg

Increased anxiety, agitation, or diaphoresis

↓

PASS = FAIL → Return to screening

↓

Does not require suctioning more than 4 h/day

President evidence of ability to protect airway (cough, gag reflex)

No evidence of upper airway obstruction in previous 48 h

No history of reintubation for excessive tracheal secretions in previous 48 h

↓

T – piecetrail (optional)

↓

PASS/FAIL → Return to screening

↓

EXTUBATE

to manage secretions, nutritional repletion, normalization of acid-base and electrolyte status, and an artificial airway of adequate size. If the aforementioned conditions are addressed, weaning may be attempted.

There are four methods of weaning. Simplest is to perform a trial of spontaneous breathing each day with a T-piece circuit providing oxygen-enriched gas. Initially brief (5–10 min), the trial can be increased in frequency and duration until the patient can breathe spontaneously for several hours. Alternatively, a single trial of up to 2h in duration is undertaken; if successful, the patient is extubated; if not, the next attempt is made on the following day. More common (and popular) are SIMV and pressure support ventilation, which are often combined. Support is decreased gradually by decreasing respiratory rate or pressure support. When combined, minimum respiratory rate is set to zero before pressure support is decreased. Pressure support of 5–8 cm H_2O is used widely to compensate for the resistance inherent in the ventilator circuit; patients who can breathe comfortably at that level should be able to be extubated. Prospective trials indicate that weaning takes up to three times longer when IMV is used rather than a spontaneous breathing trial. Approximately 10–20% of patients require re-intubation, and affected patients have mortality that is six-fold higher. Use of non-invasive ventilation after extubation may improve the likelihood of successful extubation.

Special Airway Considerations

Unplanned extubation: Patient self-extubation is a morbid event that occurs in approximately 10% of patients undergoing mechanical ventilation. Risk factors include chronic respiratory failure, poor fixation of the airway device, orotracheal intubation (which is decidedly uncomfortable), and inadequate sedation. The associated complications include re-intubation (required in one-half of such patients), ventilator-associated pneumonia, vocal cord trauma, and rarely loss of the airway with attendant cardiovascular and neurologic complications. Re-intubation is more likely in the setting of accidental intubation, decreased mentation, occurrence outside a process of active weaning, and $PaO_2{:}F_IO_2 < 200$. The risk of unplanned extubation can be decreased by appropriate sedation, vigilance during positioning of the patient and during bedside procedures, proper fixation of the airway device, and daily screening and assessment of patient readiness for liberation from the ventilator.

Re-intubation: Approximately 20% of patients require re-intubation, even if protocols are followed, and the patient meets all criteria for extubation. The rate varies widely among units; a rate that is "too low" may imply that patients are not being weaned aggressively enough, whereas a rate that is "too high" may reflect a high proportion of patients with neurologic impairment who are at highest risk. Paradoxically, use of weaning protocols, which liberate patients from mechanical ventilation sooner are associated with lesser rates of re-intubation. Re-intubation may reflect severity of illness with substantially increased risks of pneumonia and death. The cause may be either airway compromise or failure of lung/chest wall mechanics (weaning failure).

Tracheostomy: It is challenging to identify patients who will not be able to be removed from the ventilator. Possible reasons include airway obstruction, anxiety or agitation (requiring heavy doses of sedatives), aspiration syndromes, alkalosis, bronchospasm, chronic obstructive pulmonary disease, critical illness polyneuropathy or other forms of neuromuscular disease, electrolyte abnormalities, heart disease, hypothyroidism, morbid obesity, nutrition (over-or under-feeding), opioids, pleural effusion (if large), pulmonary edema, and sepsis.

The timing of tracheostomy remains controversial. There is no consensus definition of when a tracheostomy is "early" (<10 days?) or "late" (>21 days?), although trends are toward earlier performance, with decreased sedation requirements and risk of ventilator-associated pneumonia, greater patient comfort, and facilitated weaning thereafter. The shorter tube decreases airway resistance and work of breathing and facilitates pulmonary toilet by suctioning. Percutaneous tracheostomy has decreased the morbidity of tracheostomy substantially. In addition, modern high-volume, low-pressure cuffs on endotracheal tubes permit translaryngeal intubation for several weeks with relative safety. Patients who are unstable hemodynamically, coagulopathic, or on high levels of PEEP may benefit from having tracheostomy postponed until they are more stable.

Selected Readings

ARDSNetwork (2000) Ventilation with lower tidal volumes as compared with traditional tidal volumes for acute lung injury and the acute respiratory distress syndrome. N Engl J Med 342:1301–1308

Arroliga A, Frutos-Vivar F, Hall J, et al. (2005) International Mechanical Ventilation Study Group. Use of sedatives and neuromuscular blockers in a cohort of patients receiving mechanical ventilation. Chest 128:496–506

Brochard L, Rauss A, Benito S, et al. (1994) Comparison of three methods of gradual withdrawal from ventilatory support during weaning from mechanical ventilation. Am J Respir Crit Care Med 150:896–903

Dodek P, Keenen S, Cook D, et al. (2004) for the Canadian Clinical Trials Group and the Canadian Critical Care Society. Evidence-based clinical guideline for the prevention of ventilator-associated pneumonia. Ann Intern Med 141:305–313

Eachempati SR, Young C, Alexander J, et al. (1999) The clinical use of an esophageal Doppler monitor for hemo-dynamic monitoring in sepsis. J Clin Monitor Comp 15:223–225

Kollef MH, Shapiro SD, Silver P, et al. (1997) A randomized, controlled trial of protocol-directed versus physician-directed weaning from mechanical ventilation. Crit Care Med 25:567–574

MacIntyre NR, Cook DJ, Ely EW Jr, et al. (2001) Evidence-based guidelines for weaning and discontinuing ventilatory support: a collective task force facilitated by the American College of Chest Physicians, the American Association for Respiratory Care, and the American College of Critical Care Medicine. Chest 120:375S–395S

National Heart, Lung, and Blood Institute Acute Respiratory Distress Syndrome (ARDS) Clinical Trials Network Wheeler AP, Bernard GP, Thompson BT, et al. (2006) Pulmonary-artery versus central venous catheter to guide treatment of acute lung injury. N Engl J Med 354:2213–2224

Pinsky MR (2003) Hemodynamic monitoring in the intensive care unit. Clin Chest Med 24:549–560

Yang KL, Tobin MJ (1991) A prospective study of indexes predicting the outcome of trials of weaning from mechanical ventilation. N Engl J Med 324:1445–1450

3
Coma and Altered Mental Status in the Surgical Critical Care Setting; Brain Death

Joshua M. Levine and M. Sean Grady

Pearls and Pitfalls

- Altered consciousness results from dysfunction of either the upper brainstem/diencephalon, or both cerebral hemispheres. Unilateral brain lesions do not cause coma except with shift of midline structures.
- Etiologies of coma may be divided into primary brain disorders – which may be either structural or nonstructural – and systemic causes, such as toxic, metabolic, and infectious encephalopathies.
- Etiologies of coma that mandate emergent diagnosis and treatment to prevent life-or brain-threatening injury include: seizures, brain infections, acute hydrocephalus, herniation, ischemic and hemorrhagic strokes, subarachnoid hemorrhage, cerebral venous sinus thrombosis, hypertensive encephalopathy, and traumatic brain injury(TBI).
- Beware of coma mimics, especially the "locked-in" syndrome, in which the patient is awake and aware of their surroundings but is paralyzed and unable to communicate.
- Neurological examination of the coma patient focuses on four elements: (1) determination of the patient's level of arousal (wakefulness), (2) examination of the eyes, (3) elicitation of motor responses and abnormal reflexes, and (4) observation of breathing patterns.

K.I. Bland et al. (eds.), *Critical Care Surgery*,
DOI 10.1007/978-1-84996-378-7_3,
© Springer-Verlag London Limited 2011

- Focal neurological signs or abnormalities of the pupillary light reflex suggest a structural cause of coma.
- Induced hypothermia should be considered in patients who are comatose after cardiac arrest.
- Prognosis of coma is based on etiology, clinical signs, and ancillary tests including electrophysiological, neuroimaging, and biochemical studies. However, determining prognosis in any given patient remains a significant challenge.
- Brain death refers to irreversible cessation of whole-brain activity and is a clinical diagnosis.
- The three cardinal features of brain death are: (1) coma, (2) absence of brainstem reflexes, and (3) apnea.

Coma and other disorders of consciousness are common in the surgical intensive care unit (ICU) and indicate a severe disturbance of cerebral function. Management of patients with disturbed consciousness is frequently difficult because there are a myriad of possible causes, many of which require urgent intervention in order to prevent irreversible brain damage. Altered mental status is a medical emergency and mandates a prompt, systematic evaluation to diagnose and treat life-or brain-threatening disorders. Brain death is defined in the USA as irreversible cessation of whole-brain activity and is discussed at the end of this chapter.

States of consciousness fall along a spectrum, with coma at one end and normal consciousness at the other. Patients who are in coma do not respond to external stimuli in a "purposeful" manner but may demonstrate reflexive behavior. Their eyes are closed and sleep–wake cycles are absent. Coma is usually prolonged – lasting for at least hours to days, but rarely permanent – progressing either to death or to a higher level of consciousness. Deterioration of normal consciousness is often designated by terms such as "confusion" or "delirium," "stupor," and "coma." These labels are imprecise and have been defined inconsistently from study to study, and even occasionally within a given study. Attempts have been made to codify criteria for coma, vegetative state, minimally conscious state, delirium, etc. These attempts, while laudable, have not yet led to universal adoption of standard terminology. For practical purposes of the ICU physician, it is therefore advisable to use descriptive terminology and validated scales, such as the Glasgow Coma Scale (GCS).

Anatomy and Pathophysiology of Altered Mental Status

The anatomic basis of consciousness is poorly understood. At a minimum, arousal is dependent on integrity of the ascending reticular activating system, a diffuse network of neurons which originate in the pons and midbrain and project to the diencephalon (thalamus and hypothalamus) and cortex. The cerebral cortex and its subcortical connections are also necessary for normal consciousness. Disturbed consciousness is therefore produced by dysfunction of the upper brainstem/diencephalon, or by global dysfunction of the cerebral hemispheres. A unilateral hemispheric lesion does not produce coma unless either it is large enough to produce significant mass-effect on the contralateral hemisphere, or there is a preexisting contralateral lesion.

Etiologies of Coma

Causes of altered mental status and coma are protean, and are divided into primary brain disorders and systemic derangements that secondarily impact brain function. Primary brain disorders may be structural abnormalities – e.g., brain infarction, hemorrhage, hydrocephalus, contusion, herniation – or they may be nonstructural disturbances, such as seizures. Systemic disturbances that cause encephalopathy include metabolic derangements, exposure to toxins, and systemic infections.

The most common causes of coma are traumatic brain injury (TBI), hypoxic-ischemic encephalopathy (HIE), drug overdose, ischemic and hemorrhagic strokes, central nervous system infections, and brain herniation from space-occupying lesions. Table 3.1 lists causes of altered mental status. A detailed discussion of these conditions is beyond the scope of this chapter; however, a few warrant special mention because rapid

TABLE 3.1. A partial list of the etiologies of coma and altered mental status (Adapted from Stevens and Bhardwaj, 2006).

I. Primary brain disorders

  (a) Structural lesions

      (i) Traumatic brain injury

        1. Diffuse axonal injury

        2. Contusions

        3. Subdural hematomas

        4. Epidural hematomas

      (ii) Cerebrovascular disorders

        1. Ischemic strokes

        2. Spontaneous intracerebral hemorrhage

        3. Subarachnoid hemorrhage

        4. Hypoxic-ischemic encephalopathy

        5. Cerebral venous sinus thrombosis

      (iii) Malignant disease

        1. Brain tumors

      (iv) Infectious diseases

        1. Brain abscesses

      (v) Demyelinating disease

        1. Acute disseminated encephalomyelitis

        2. Central pontine myelinolysis

      (vi) Hydrocephalus

  (b) Nonstructural disorders

      (i) Infectious diseases

        1. Bacterial meningoencephalitis

(continued)

TABLE 3.1. (continued)

    2. Carcinomatous or lymphomatous meningitis

    3. Viral encephalitis

  (ii) Generalized seizures, status epilepticus

  (iii) Basilar migraines

II. Systemic disorders

  (a) Toxic encephalopathies

    (i) Medication overdose

      1. Opioids, benzodiazepines, barbiturates, tricyclics, etc.

    (ii) Illicit drug exposure

      1. Opioids, alcohols, amphetamines, etc.

    (iii) Environmental toxin exposure

      1. Carbon monoxide

      2. Heavy metals

      3. Pesticides

  (b) Metabolic encephalopathies

    (i) Hypoglycemia, hyperglycemia

    (ii) Hyponatremia, hypernatremia

    (iii) Hypercalcemia

    (iv) Hepatic encephalopathy

    (v) Uremia

    (vi) Vitamin deficiencies (thiamine, niacin)

    (vii) Hypothermia, severe hyperthermia

    (viii) Hypothyroidism, hyperthyroidism

    (ix) Urea cycle disorders

  (c) Infections

    (i) Urinary tract infections

    (ii) Pneumonia

    (iii) Sepsis

diagnosis and urgent treatment are essential in order to limit permanent brain injury. These include seizures, brain infections, acute hydrocephalus, herniation, ischemic and hemorrhagic strokes, subarachnoid hemorrhage, cerebral venous sinus thrombosis, hypertensive encephalopathy, and TBI.

Differential Diagnosis (Mimics) of Coma and the Vegetative State

Patients may become unresponsive from conditions that mimic coma or a vegetative state. In the locked-in syndrome, destruction of the ventral pons leaves the patient quadriplegic and mute. Patients are often aware of their surroundings and may communicate only through vertical eye movements and blinking, which are spared. With more rostral pontine lesions, vertical eye movements and blinking are lost. In this state, akin to receiving a neuromuscular blocking agent without a sedative, the patient has no means of communication. Severe Guillain-Barre syndrome, botulism, and critical illness neuropathy may similarly result in complete de-efferentation. Catatonia is a manifestation of severe psychiatric illness in which patients open their eyes, do not speak or follow commands, and may exhibit waxy flexibility. The remainder of the neurological exam and the electroencephalogram (EEG) are normal. Akinetic mutism, due to bilateral medial frontal lobe injury, is a profound form of abulia (lack of motivation), in which patients are unable to speak or to move but open their eyes and may track visual stimuli.

Clinical Approach to the Comatose Patient

Overview

Evaluation and management of the comatose patient requires an emergent and structured approach (Fig. 3.1). As with all medical emergencies, attention is first directed toward

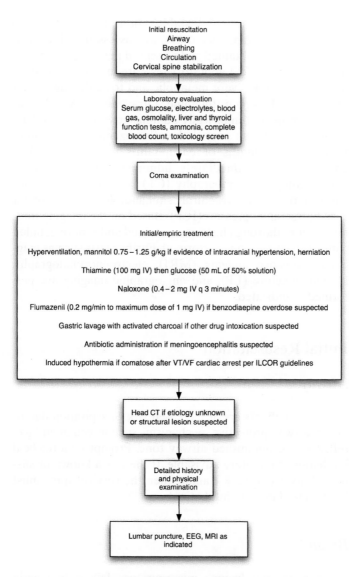

FIGURE 3.1. Algorithm for initial approach to the comatose patient (Adapted from Stevens and Bhardwaj, 2006).

patient resuscitation and stabilization. Respiratory and hemodynamic parameters are rapidly assessed and normalized. A history is obtained and a focused neurological examination is performed. Laboratory tests are sent to evaluate for infection and for severe metabolic and toxic derangements. Supplemental oxygen, thiamine, intravenous (IV) glucose, and naloxone are empirically administered. If a benzodiazepine overdose is suspected, then flumazenil may be administered. If meningitis or encephalitis is suspected, then antibiotics are immediately administered. Noncontrast cranial computed tomography (CT) is obtained to further confirm orexcludeastructurallesion,andtolookforsignsofincreasedintracranial pressure(ICP). Based on the imaging findings, a more thorough history is obtained and a more detailed clinical examination is performed. Further tests such as magnetic resonance imaging (MRI), electroencephalography, lumbar puncture (LP), and angiographic imaging are performed as indicated.

Initial Resuscitation

Airway

Comatose patients are at increased risk of aspiration due to loss of airway-protective mechanisms such as cough and gag reflexes, and diminished airway tone. Prompt endotracheal intubation is therefore advisable. If there is a known or suspected history of neck trauma, then the cervical spine must be stabilized prior to intubation.

Breathing

Hypercapnic and hypoxe micrespiratory failure frequently accompany coma and should be treated with prompt mechanical ventilation. Injuries to the brain stem and spinal cord may cause abnormal respiratory patterns or complete loss of respiratory drive. Aspiration of gastric contents and prolonged ventilatory failure are common causes of hypoxemia. On occasion, hypoxemia results from neurogenic pulmonary edema.

Circulation

Cardiac arrhythmias may be seen when coma occurs from global ischemia in the setting of myocardial infarction, or pulmonary or fat embolism. Rarely, arrhythmias may result from primary neurological injury. Arrhythmias should be treated according to standard advanced cardiac life support (ACLS) protocols.

Severe hypertension frequently accompanies coma. When coma is accompanied by reduced cerebral blood flow, as occurs with increased ICP or basilar artery thrombosis, hypertension is a compensatory response aimed at restoration of cerebral perfusion pressure. In this situation, aggressive lowering of blood pressure may precipitate cerebral infarction. If, however, coma is the result of severe hypertension, as in hypertensive encephalopathy, then blood pressure must be lowered emergently. It is difficult to distinguish on clinical grounds whether hypertension is the cause or an effect of the underlying problem. In either case, blood pressure should only be lowered if there is clear evidence of end-organ damage (heart failure, kidney failure, hypertensive encephalopathy). IV agents such as labetolol or nicardipine should be titrated to lower the mean arterial pressure by no more than 20%. Nitroprusside may increase ICP and should be used with caution. It is imperative to monitor neurological function for signs of ischemia while blood pressure is being lowered.

Hypotension in the setting of coma is usually due to systemic causes, such as cardiac dysfunction, sepsis, or hemorrhage. Blood pressure should be restored to baseline with isotonic IV fluids and, if necessary, pressors. Hypertonic fluids may be used for volume resuscitation in patients with hypovolemic shock and TBI. Hypotonic fluids may exacerbate brain edema by lowering serum osmolarity and should not be administered. The cause of the hypotension should be sought and rapidly corrected.

History

In many cases, for example, after trauma or cardiac arrest, the cause of the coma is evident. In other cases, clues must be sought from the history. Family members and witnesses must be interviewed about the time course of the illness, preexisting medical conditions, medication history, suicidal behavior, and illicit drug use.

Neurological Assessment

By allowing the examiner to localize the lesion, the initial neurological examination helps to narrow the list of etiological possibilities. For example, integrity of brainstem function and absence of focal signs suggests a toxic or metabolic disorder. In contrast, asymmetric findings and brainstem dysfunction are more consistent with a structural etiology. The exam is also used to exclude conditions which mimic coma. Serial examinations of the comatose patient over time are essential and provide information about efficacy of treatment, worsening of the primary process, and prognosis.

The coma examination is focused on four elements: (1) determination of the patient's level of arousal (wakefulness), (2) examination of the eyes, (3) elicitation of motor responses and abnormal reflexes, and (4) observation of breathing patterns.

1. *Level of Consciousness*

   First, the patient should be observed. Patients who exhibit spontaneous eyes opening, verbalization attempts, moaning, tossing, reaching, leg crossing, yawning, coughing, or swallowing have a higher level of consciousness than those who do not. The examiner should next assess the patient's response to a series of stimuli which escalate in intensity. The patient's name should be called loudly. If there is no response, the examiner should stimulate the patient by gently shaking him. If this produces no response, the examiner must use a noxious stimulus, such as pressure to the supraorbital ridge, nail beds, or sternum, or nasal tickle with a cotton wisp. Responses such as grimacing, eye opening, grunting, or verbalization should be documented. Motor responses provide information not only about sensation and limb strength, but also about level of consciousness. The examiner should note whether stimuli produce "purposeful" or non-stereotyped limb movements – such as reaching toward the site of stimulation ("localization"). This implies a degree of intact cortical function. Stereotyped limb movements are generally mediated by brain and spinal reflexes and do not require cortical input. Examples include extension and internal rotation of the limbs (decerebrate posturing), upper extremity flexion (decorticate posturing), and flexion at the ankle, knee, and hip ("triple-flexion").

2. *Eye Examination*

In coma, the neuro-ophthalmological examination focuses on (a) the pupils, (b) resting eye position and eye movements, (c) appearance of the retina, and (d) the corneal reflex.

(a) *Pupillary examination*: Pupillary size, shape, and reactivity to light should be assessed. In general, abnormalities of the pupillary light reflex suggest a structural abnormality. However, certain drugs may also affect the pupillary light reflex. Metabolic causes of coma typically do not affect the pupils. The pupils are normally round, have equal diameters, and briskly constrict when illuminated. When unequal pupils (anisocoria) are observed, it is important to establish whether it is the larger or the smaller pupil that is abnormal. This is accomplished by examining the eyes both in the light and in the dark. When the lights are extinguished, an abnormally small pupil will fail to dilate fully and the degree of anisocoria will increase. In contrast, when the abnormal pupil is the larger one, the degree of anisocoria will be maximal under full illumination when the larger pupil fails to constrict fully. In the ICU, the most important causes of a unilaterally dilated pupil are compressive lesions of the oculomotor nerve complex, such as uncal herniation and intracranial aneurysms. A complete third nerve palsy results in ipsilateral mydriasis, inferolateral deviation of the eye, and a severe ipsilateral ptosis. The most important cause of unilateral small pupil is the Horner's syndrome, which consists of miosis and mild ipsilateral ptosis. Depending on the location of the lesion, ipsilateral facial anhidrosis may also be present. Bilaterally fixed and dilated pupils are seen in the terminal stages of brain death but also with anticholinergic medications, such as atropine. Hyperadrenergic states (e.g., pain, anxiety, cocaine intoxication) produce bilaterally large and reactive pupils. Reactive pinpoint(<1 mm) pupils are observed with opiate and barbiturate intoxication, and after extensive pontine injury.

(b) *Resting eye position and eye movements*: Eye position and spontaneous movements should be noted. Horizontal or vertical misalignment of the eyes as well as spontaneous roving or rhythmic and repetitive vertical movements should be documented. The frontal lobe cortex (frontal eye fields) mediates conjugate deviation of the eyes toward the contralateral side. Lateral deviation of both eyes therefore indicates a destructive lesion in the ipsilateral frontal lobe or an excitatory focus (seizure) in the contralateral hemisphere. A destructive unilateral pontine lesion, and rarely, a thalamic lesion, will cause conjugate deviation to the contralateral side. Downward deviation of the eyes is caused by dysfunction of the dorsal midbrain and is seen with hydrocephalus, tumors, and strokes. Dysconjugate gaze is frequently seen in sedated patients and usually represents unmasking of a latent esophoria or exophoria. Roving, or slow to-and-fro eye movements, implies functional integrity of the brainstem. Ocular bobbing – fast conjugate downward gaze followed by a slow upward correction to midposition – implies extensive pontine injury. Ocular dipping – slow conjugate down gaze followed by fast upward gaze – also localizes to the pons. With a skew deviation, one eye is higher than the other, and the lesion is usually in the midbrain on the side of the higher eye, or in the pontomedullary junction on side of the lower eye. In the critically ill comatose patients, there is a high incidence of nonconvulsive seizures and jerking movements of the eyes may be the only evidence of seizure activity. If spontaneous eye movements are absent, then an oculocephalic response ("doll's eyes") should be sought by turning the head horizontally and vertically. This maneuver should not be performed on trauma patients with known or suspected cervical spine instability. Normally the eyes move opposite to the direction of head turning. Testing the oculocephalic response may uncover a vertical gaze paresis, a skew deviation, or a sixth nerve palsy that was not otherwise obvious.

If an oculocephalic response cannot be elicited, then anoculovestibular ("cold-caloric") response is sought. First, the tympanic membrane should be visualized to ensure that it is intact and unobstructed. The head of the bed should be set at 30° to align the patient's horizontal semicircular canals perpendicular to the floor. Then, using an angiocatheter or a butterfly catheter without the needle, 30–60 ml of ice-cold water is instilled into the external auditory canal against the tympanic membrane. This inhibits the ipsilateral vestibular system and normally causes the eyes first to move slowly toward the ipsilateral ear and then to jerk quickly toward the contralateral ear. The initial slow response is mediated by the unopposed contralateral vestibular system in the brainstem, and the subsequent corrective nystagmus is mediated by the frontal eye fields. With bilateral cortical dysfunction and an intact brainstem, slow tonic deviation of the eyes toward the ipsilateral ear is observed and is not followed by contralateral nystagmus. In early metabolic coma, the oculocephalic and oculovestibular responses are preserved. Absent responses indicate diffuse brainstem dysfunction and are seen in primary brainstem injury, late transtentorial herniation, barbiturate intoxication, and brain death.

(c) *Retinal examination*: A fundoscopic examination should be performed to look for signs of intracranial hypertension. Papilledema is swelling of the optic nerve head from elevated ICP. It is almost always bilateral and may be accompanied by retinal hemorrhages, exudates, cotton wool spots, and ultimately by enlargement of the optic cup. Papilledema develops over hours to days. Its absence, therefore, does not imply normal ICP, especially in the acute setting. Pulsatility of the retinal veins strongly suggests normal ICP. Terson's syndrome is vitreous, subhyaloid, or retinal hemorrhage associated with subarachnoid hemorrhage.

(d) *The corneal reflex*: The corneal reflex is tested by gently touching the cornea of each eye with a drop of saline or a cotton wisp and observing for eyelid closure. Failure of unilateral eyelid closure suggests facial nerve dysfunction on that side. Failure of bilateral eyelid closure with stimulation of one cornea, but not the other, implies trigeminal nerve dysfunction on the stimulated side. Failure of bilateral eyelid closure upon stimulation of either cornea usually implies pontine dysfunction.

Motor Responses and Abnormal Reflexes

The symmetry of motor responses and reflexes, and the presence of abnormal movements often allow discrimination between structural and systemic etiologies of altered mental status. First, the patient should be observed for any abnormal or spontaneous movements. Asterixis implies a metabolic disturbance such as uremia or hepatic encephalopathy. Twitching or jerking of the face or limbs, even if subtle, raises the suspicion for seizures. Asymmetry of resting-limb position is frequently a subtle sign of weakness. For example, a paretic leg will lie externally rotated. Next, the patient is stimulated and the examiner must search for asymmetry in the patient's face (grimace) and appendicular motor responses. A less vigorous response on one side of the body indicates a contralateral structural lesion involving the motor pathways above the level of the caudal medulla. Paraparesis and quadriparesis raise the possibility of spinal cord injury, especially in the setting of trauma.

Breathing Patterns

A variety of breathing patterns may be observed in coma. Although these may yield clues regarding the location of the intracranial lesion, in clinical practice, breathing patterns are often obscured by the use of sedatives, paralytics, and mechanical ventilation. Apneustic respirations are characterized by a prolonged end-inspiratory pause. This pattern may be seen after focal injury to the dorsal lower half of the pons (e.g., stroke), but may also be observed with meningitis, hypoxia, and hypoglycemia. Cluster breathing consists of several rapid, shallow breaths followed by a prolonged pause, and localizes to the upper medulla. Ataxic respirations, or Biot's breathing, is a chaotic pattern in which the length and depth of the inspiratory and expiratory phases are irregular. It may occur after injury to the respiratory centers in the lower medulla. Apnea may be seen in a variety of neurological and non-neurological disorders and is of no localizing value. Kussmaul respirations are rapid, deep breaths that usually signal metabolic acidosis, but also may be observed with pontomesencephalic lesions. Cheyne-Stokes respiration refers to alternating spells of apnea and crescendo-decrescendo hyperpnea. It has minimal value in localization and is seen with diffuse cerebral injury, hypoxia, hypocapnea, and congestive heart failure. Agonal gasps reflect bilateral lower medullary injury and are seen in the terminal stages of brain injury.

The Glasgow Coma Scale

The GCS (Table 3.2) is a useful tool for the initial neurological survey. It was initially intended for use in TBI; however, it is now a widely accepted tool for evaluation of consciousness in the general critically ill population. It may be performed

TABLE 3.2. Glasgow Coma Scale (Adapted from Teasdale and Jennett, 1974. Copyright 1974, with permission from Elsevier).

Motor response	
Follows commands	6
Localizes pain	5
Withdraws to pain	4
Flexion	3
Extension	2
None	1
Verbal response	
Oriented	5
Confused speech	4
Inappropriate words	3
Incomprehensible	2
None	1
Eye opening	
Spontaneous	4
To command	3
To pain	2
None	1

quickly and reliably at the bedside. GCS score predicts survival and neurological outcome in TBI, nontraumatic coma, ischemic stroke, intracerebral hemorrhage, subarachnoid hemorrhage, and meningitis. It also predicts mortality in the general critical-care patient. The GCS has limitations. It is a relatively crude instrument that is insensitive to subtle variations in mental status. A given score in the mid-range (6–12) may be assigned to patients with significantly different degrees of impaired consciousness through different combinations of scores in each of the three categories. The GCS has limited utility in patients with aphasia, significant facial trauma, or in those who are sedated or intubated. Despite its limitations, the GCS is a mainstay of clinical assessment that aids in communication, prognostication, and research. The Full Outline of UnResponsiveness (FOUR) score is a new coma scale that incorporates brainstem reflexes and breathing patterns (Fig. 3.2). It is simple, recognizes brain death, uncal herniation, and the locked-in state, and has comparable inter-rater reliability to the GCS. Whether this scale gains widespread acceptance remains to be seen.

Laboratory Investigations

Metabolic and toxic encephalopathies account for a significant proportion of altered mental status. Commonly encountered metabolic disturbances include severe hypernatremia and hyponatremia, hypercalcemia, elevated blood urea nitrogen, hyperammonemia, hypoglycemia and hyperglycemia, hypercarbia, hypoxemia, and severe hyperthyroidism and hypothyroidism. A toxicology screen detects exposure to common drugs and toxins. Plasma osmolality should be measured so that the plasma osmolal gap may be determined. The osmolal gap is the difference between the calculated osmolarity ($2[Na] + [BUN]/2.8 + [glucose]/18$) and the measured osmolality. The osmolal gap is elevated with intoxication from alcohols, such as methanol, and ethylene glycol. A complete blood count should be obtained to help assess for an infectious cause of encephalopathy.

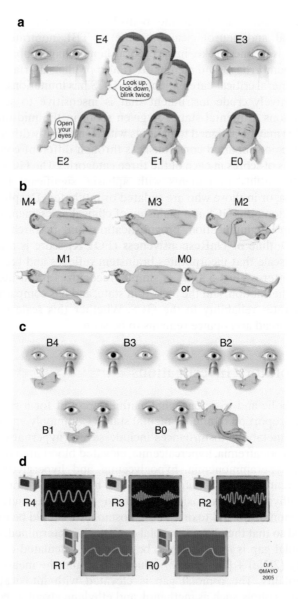

FIGURE 3.2. The FOUR score. Instructions for the assessment of the individual categories of the FOUR (Full Outline of UnResponsiveness) score. (**a**) For eye response (**e**), grade the best possible

FIGURE 3.2. (continued) response after at least three trials in an attempt to elicit the best level of alertness. A score of E4 indicates at least three voluntary excursions. If eyelids are closed, the examiner should open them and examine tracking of a finger or object. Tracking with the opening of one eyelid will suffice in cases of eyelid edema or facial trauma. If tracking is absent horizontally, examine vertical tracking. Alternatively, two blinks on command should be documented. This will recognize a locked-in syndrome (patient is fully aware). A score of E3 indicates the absence of voluntary tracking with open eyes. A score of E2 indicates eyelids opening to a loud voice. A score of E1 indicates eyelids open to pain stimulus. A score of E0 indicates no eyelid opening to pain. (**b**) For motor response (M), grade the best possible response of the arms. A score of M4 indicates that the patient demonstrated at least one of three hand positions (thumbs-up, fist, or peace sign) with either hand. A score of M3 (localization) indicates that the patient touched the examiner's hand after a painful stimulus compressing the temporomandibular joint or supraorbital nerve. A score of M2 indicates any flexion movement of the upper limbs. A score of M1 indicates extensor response to pain. A score of M0 indicates no motor response to pain, or myoclonus status epilepticus. (**c**) For brainstem reflexes (**b**), grade the best possible response. Examine pupillary and corneal reflexes. Preferably, corneal reflexes are tested by instilling two to three drops sterile saline on the cornea from a distance of 4–6 in. (this minimizes corneal trauma from repeated examinations). Sterile cotton swabs can also be used. The cough reflex to tracheal suctioning is tested only when both of these reflexes are absent. A score of B4 indicates pupil and corneal reflexes are present. A score of B3 indicates one pupil wide and fixed. A score of B2 indicates either pupil or cornea reflexes are absent. A score of B1 indicates both pupil and cornea reflexes are absent. A score of B0 indicates pupil, cornea, and cough reflex (using tracheal suctioning) are absent. (**d**) For respiration (R), determine spontaneous breathing pattern in a nonintubated patient and grade simply as regular (R4), or irregular (R2), Cheyne-Stokes (R3) breathing. In mechanically ventilated patients, assess the pressure waveform of spontaneous respiratory pattern or the patient triggering of the ventilator (R1). The ventilator monitor displaying respiratory patterns can be used to identify the patient-generated breaths on the ventilator. No adjustments are made to the ventilator while the patient is graded, but grading is done preferably with PaCO2 within normal limits. A standard apnea (oxygen-diffusion) test may be needed when patient breathes at ventilator rate (R0) (Reprinted from Wijdicks et al., 2005. With permission).

Initial Therapy

Initial therapy of the comatose patient is often empiric. If signs or symptoms of increased ICP or herniation are detected, mannitol is administered as a 1 gm/kg IV bolus. Hyperventilation causes cerebral vasoconstriction, which reduces cerebral blood volume and hence lowers ICP. While extremely effective, the effect on ICP is short-lived and hyperventilation may cause cerebral ischemia. Hyperventilation should therefore only be used emergently for a short period of time as a bridge to more definitive (usually surgical) therapy. Rarely, thiamine deficiency may cause profound alterations in consciousness and all patients should receive IV thiamine. Glucose is administered if serum glucose is less than 60 mg/dl or cannot immediately be measured. In patients with very low thiamine stores, glucose administration may theoretically precipitate acute thiamine deficiency.

Therefore, glucose should be administered after thiamine. Naloxone is empirically given to reverse opiate intoxication. Routine empiric administration of flumazenil is controversial and should be given only when the history suggests a benzodiazepine overdose. If another toxic ingestion is suspected, then gastric lavage with activated charcoal is appropriate. Bacterial meningitis and herpes simplex encephalitis are associated with high mortality rates if not treated expeditiously. When brain infection is suspected, treatment with antibiotics should occur right away. If a head CT and LP cannot be performed immediately, then antibiotic administration should precede these diagnostic tests. Convincing evidence suggests that patients who are comatose after resuscitation from out-of-hospital cardiac arrest due to ventricular fibrillation (VF) should be cooled to 32–34C for 12–24 h. It is reasonable to generalize this strategy to patients with in-hospital cardiac arrest and to those with pulseless electrical activity.

Neuroimaging Studies

Noncontrast cranial CT is indicated in all new cases of unexplained coma and is the test of first choice. CT rapidly identifies intra-and extra-axial cerebral hemorrhages, brain herniation, cerebral edema, and hydrocephalus. MRI is indicated in patients whose coma remains unexplained after CT. MRI has a higher sensitivity than CT for acute ischemic stroke, intracerebral hemorrhage, inflammatory conditions, brain abscesses, brain tumors, cerebral edema, cerebral venous sinus thrombosis, and diffuse axonal injury. MRI is less widely available than CT, is more time-consuming, and requires non-ferromagnetic equipment, making it less feasible for many critically ill patients. The risks of transporting patients to the CT or MRI scanner, and the time it takes to complete the studies must be weighed against the benefit of the information they may yield.

Prognosis of the Comatose Patient

Coma, by definition, is self-limited. Survivors may recover to a persistent vegetative state, to complete neurological recovery, or to an intermediate state of neurological disability. The Glasgow Outcome Scale (GOS) is an established metric of recovery (Table 3.3). Although it fails to capture the full breadth of possible neurological outcomes, it is widely used by clinical investigators for traumatic and nontraumatic coma.

Determining the prognosis of comatose patients poses a significant challenge. Studies that have addressed the prognosis of coma are plagued by numerous problems that limit their clinical applicability. First, coma has been defined inconsistently across studies. Second, virtually all studies involved patients in whom care was intentionally limited, leading to a "self-fulfilling prophecy" bias. Third, most studies were performed prior to major advances in intensive care, such as induced hypothermia and intensive insulin therapy, which have been shown to improve outcome in certain patient populations. Last, studies have not yet systematically addressed the impact of clinical confounders such as metabolic disturbances, sedative and paralytic medications, and shock.

Prognosis of coma is based on etiology, clinical signs, and ancillary tests including electrophysiological, neuroimaging, and biochemical studies. As a general rule, coma due to closed head injury has a better prognosis than nontraumatic coma. Coma due to penetrating head injury is associated with a poor prognosis. It is probably also true that in cases of nontraumatic coma, nonstructural etiologies are associated with a better prognosis than structural etiologies.

For nontraumatic coma, the best evidence regarding the utility of clinical signs and ancillary tests for prognosis comes from studies of survivors of cardiac arrest. These data are summarized in a practice parameter that was recently issued by the Quality Standards Subcommittee of the American Academy of Neurology. Based on their findings, clinical signs that most accurately portend poor prognosis include myoclonic status epilepticus within the first 24 h after primary circulatory arrest, absence of pupillary responses within days 1–3 after cardiopulmonary resuscitation (CPR), absence of corneal reflexes within days 1–3 after CPR, and absence of extensor motor responses after day 3. Although certain electroencephalographic patterns, such as burst suppression and generalized epileptiform discharges are associated with poor prognosis, EEG lacks sufficient prognostic accuracy and is not recommended as a tool for predicting outcome. Somatosensory evoked potentials (SSEPs) are more useful for prognostication. SSEP is less susceptible than EEG to the confounding effects of drugs and metabolic derangement. Bilateral absence of the N20 component of the SSEP with median nerve stimulation after day 1 most accurately predicts poor prognosis. Numerous serum and cerebrospinal fluid (CSF) biomarkers have been studied for their prognostic value. To date, the only marker with sufficient prognostic accuracy to be recommended is neuron-specific enolase (NSE). Serum NSE levels of >33 mg/l on days 1–3 strongly predict poor outcome; however, this test is not yet widely available. Ongoing studies are addressing the prognostic role of cranial CT, MRI, and magnetic resonance spectroscopy.

Studies to determine prognosis of traumatic coma are inherently difficult. Closed head injury affects a heterogeneous patient population, encompasses a variety of structural brain lesions, and is often accompanied by systemic trauma and major systemic derangements. A handful of factors have been identified that are associated with poor prognosis. These include advanced age, a low initial GCS score, the presence of diffuse axonal injury on neuroimaging studies, and the presence of hypoxia or hypotension. Genetic markers may ultimately prove useful in determining prognosis. Recently, investigators determined that patients possessing the apoE4 allele have a worse outcome after TBI.

Brain Death

Brain death refers to irreversible cessation of whole-brain activity. The concept of brain death was established in the 1950s and diagnostic criteria were first published in 1968. The idea that brain death is legally equivalent to cardiac death has since gained widespread acceptance in the USA and in many Western countries and has greatly facilitated organ donation.

Brain death is a clinical diagnosis that rests on the demonstration of (1) deep coma, (2) absence of brainstem reflexes, and (3) apnea. In an attempt to standardize diagnostic criteria, the American Academy of Neurology published a practice parameter in 1995. However, variations in practice exist across institutions, and physicians who determine brain death must be familiar with the specific protocol used in their hospital.

Prior to the determination of brain death, the physician should establish an irreversible cause of brain failure based on clinical and/or neuroimaging evidence. Medical conditions which might confound the neurological exam – such as hypothermia, severe metabolic or endocrine derangements, hypotension, and drug intoxication – must be excluded or corrected. In general, two clinical examinations, separated by a period of hours, are performed, followed by an apnea test. Coma is demonstrated by the lack of cerebral motor responses to pain in all four extremities. Patients should not grimace to pain.

The following brainstem reflexes must be absent: pupillary light reflex, oculocephalic reflex (tested only in patients without cervical spine trauma); oculovestibular reflex, corneal reflex; cough with deep tracheal suctioning; and gag. Prior to apnea testing, the partial pressures of arterial oxygen and carbon dioxide (pCO_2) should be normalized. The patient is disconnected from the ventilator for at least 8 min and observed for respiratory movements. pCO_2 is then measured and the patient is reconnected to the ventilator. Absence of respiratory movements and either a $pCO_2 > 60$ mmHg ora rise in $pCO_2 > 20$ mmHg above baseline constitutes a positive test (consistent with brain death). The apnea test should be terminated immediately if hemodynamic instability or hypoxemia occurs.

Ancillary tests to confirm brain death need not be performed on a routine basis and are used when conditions exist that interfere with the clinical assessment, such as severe facial trauma, preexisting pupillary abnormalities, and toxic levels of certain medications. These tests fall into two categories, electrophysiological tests – EEG and SSEP, and cerebral blood flow studies – including conventional angiography, transcranial Doppler ultrasonography, and technetium-99 m nuclear blood flow scans. Guidelines exist for the performance and interpretation of each type of study.

Conclusions

Altered mental status and coma occur commonly in the surgical ICU. Physicians should develop an efficient diagnostic approach that facilitates rapid treatment in order to minimize additional brain injury. The clinical exam, laboratory tests, and neuroimaging studies are powerful tools that help to determine whether a structural or systemic abnormality exists, thus narrowing the differential diagnosis. Currently there are few widely available means of reliably determining prognosis in coma¬tose patients. Genetic and metabolic markers and advanced neuroimaging modalities may ultimately prove helpful.

Selected Readings

Bernard SA, Gary TW, Buirt MD, et al. (2002) Treatment of comatose survivors of out-of-hospital cardiac arrest with induced hypothermia. New Engl J Med 346:557–563

Jennett B, Bond M (1975) Assessment of outcome after severe brain damage. Lancet 1:480–484

The Hypothermia After Cardiac Arrest (HACA) study group (2002) Mild therapeutic hypothermia to improve the neurologic outcome after cardiac arrest. New Engl J Med 346:549–556

Levy DE, Caronna JJ, Singer BH, et al. (1985) Predicting outcome from hypoxic-ischemic coma. JAMA 253:1420–1426

Nolan JP, Morley PT, Vanden Hoek TL, et al. (2003) Therapeutic hypothermia after cardiac arrest. An advisory statement by the Advanced Life Support Task Force of the International Liaison Committee on Resuscitation. Circulation 108:118–121

Plum F, Posner JB (1980) The diagnosis of stupor and coma, 3rd edn. FA Davis, Philadelphia, PA

Report of the Quality Standards Subcommittee of the American Academy of Neurology (1995) Practice para-meters for determining brain death in adults (Summary statement). Neurology 45(5):1012–1014

Stevens RD, Bhardwaj A (2006) Approach to the comatose patient. Crit Care Med 34(1):31–41

Teasdale G, Jennett B (1974) Assessment of coma and impaired consciousness. A practical scale. Lancet 2:81–84

Wijdicks EF, Bamlet WR, Maramattom BV, et al. (2005) Validation of a new coma scale: the FOUR score. Annals Neurol 58:585–593

Wijdicks EF, Hijdra A, Young GB, et al. (2006) Practice Wijdicks EF, Kokmen E, O'Brien PC (1998) Measurement parameter: prediction of outcome in comatose survivors of impaired consciousness in the neurological intensive after cardiopulmonary resuscitation (an evidence-based care unit: a new test. J Neurol, Neurosurg Psychiatr review). Neurology 67:203–210 64:117–119

4
Management of Cardiac Arrhythmias

Rebecca C. Britt and L.D. Britt

Pearls and Pitfalls

- All arrhythmias are caused by abnormal automaticity, reentry, or a combination of both.
- Narrow complex tachyarrhythmia is defined by a heart rate greater than 100 beats/min with a QRS duration of 120 ms or less as demonstrated on EKG or monitor.
- Wide complex tachyarrhythmia is defined by a heart rate greater than 100 beats/min with a prolonged QRS complex of greater than 120 ms and originates from either a supraventricular or ventricular focus.
- For tachyarrhythmias in the hemodynamically unstable patient, direct current (DC) cardioversion is the treatment option of choice to restore sinus rhythm.
- In the hemodynamically stable patient with atrial fibrillation, treatment strategies include rate control, termination of the atrial fibrillation with maintenance of sinus rhythm, and antiembolic therapy.
- Patients with unstable ventricular tachycardia and ventricular fibrillation should be treated with defibrillation.
- Amiodarone 150 mg IV bolus is the treatment of choice for hemodynamically stable patients with monomorphic ventricular tachycardia.

K.I. Bland et al. (eds.), *Critical Care Surgery*,
DOI 10.1007/978-1-84996-378-7_4,
© Springer-Verlag London Limited 2011

Introduction

Cardiac arrhythmias are common in the general population and occur frequently in the early postoperative period. While the majority are not clinically significant, transient arrhythmias in the perioperative period are reported as frequently as 60% of the time. A study of 4,181 patients who were in sinus rhythm at the time of initial preoperative evaluation, found perioperative supraventricular arrhythmias in about 8% of patients. These perioperative arrhythmias were associated with a 33% increase in duration of stay.

Anatomy and Physiology

The sinoatrial (SA) node, which lies beneath the junction of the superior vena cava and the right atrial appendage, is supplied by the sinus node artery, which arises from the right or circumflex coronary artery. The atrioventricular (AV) node, which sits on the right atrial side of the AV septum, receives its blood supply from the posterior descending coronary artery. No specific conduction path has been identified from the SA to the AV node. The bundle of His begins at the AV node and usually descends on the left side of the ventricular septum and branches into the left and right bundles just below the aortic valve. The left bundle branch supplies the ventricular septum as well as the anteroseptal and postero-medial papillary muscles. The right bundle supplies the medial papillary muscle as well as the right ventricular wall.

The SA and AV nodes both exhibit automaticity and fire spontaneously. Normal heartbeats originate in the SA node and lead to depolarization through the right and left atria followed by atrial contraction. This impulse stimulates the AV node and the bundle of His, thereby transmitting depolarization waves to the right and left His-Purkinje fibers and thus depolarizes the ventricular wall, leading to ventricular contraction.

All arrhythmias are caused by either abnormal automaticity, reentry, or a combination of both. Abnormal automaticity occurs when pathologic conditions move the resting membrane potential towards threshold, allowing for hyperexcitable, "irritable" cardiac muscle. Normal cardiac muscle has a long refractory period such that few myocytes remain excitable at the end of a beat. Myocardial ischemia, fibrosis, and necrosis lead to slowing of myocardial conduction, such that surrounding fibers may be past the refractory period when the impulse leaves the damages area, which leads to abnormal impulse stimulation with formation of a reentrant circuit.

Etiology

Risk factors for development of supraventricular arrhythmias include age greater than 70 years, preoperative congestive heart failure, and performance of abdominal, thoracic, or major vascular operations. Perioperative ventricular arrhythmias are increased in patients with preoperative ventricular ectopy, congestive heart failure, and smoking. Hypoxia, hypercarbia, hypokalemia, acid-base disorders, acute volume depletion, and myocardial infarction also contribute to the development of arrhythmias.

Clinical Presentation

Continuous electrocardiographic monitoring in the perioperative period leads to the detection of many arrhythmias. Bradycardia, defined by a heart rate less than 60 beats/min, can be normal or abnormal. Tachyarrhythmias, defined by a heart rate greater than 100 beats/min, are divided further into narrow and wide QRS complex tachyarrhythmias. Patients will complain frequently of palpitations and a sense that their heart is racing in the setting of a tachyarrhythmia. Hemodynamic instability may be associated with these arrhythmia.

Narrow complex tachyarrhythmia is defined by a heart rate of greater than 100 beats/min with a QRS duration of 120 ms or less. The site of origin for narrow complex tachycardias is supraventricular with normal conduction through the bundle of His and Purkinje fibers. Examples include sinus tachycardia, supraventricular tachycardia, atrial fibrillation, and atrial flutter.

Wide complex tachyarrhythmia, defined by a heart rate of greater than 100 beats/min with a prolonged QRS complex greater than 120 ms, originates from either a supraventricular or ventricular focus. The accurate diagnosis of wide complex tachyarrhythmias is crucial, because immediate treatment is required frequently; delayed or inappropriate treatment can be dangerous. Examples of wide complex arrhythmias include ventricular tachycardia (VT), Torsades de Pointes, and ventricular fibrillation.

The initial approach to a patient with arrhythmia is to determine whether the patient is experiencing signs and symptoms related to the rapid heart rate. Symptoms include hypotension, shock, shortness of breath, chest pain, and decreased level of consciousness. If the patient has clinically significant hemodynamic instability, an attempt at cardioversion should be made. Important history should include whether the patient has a history of cardiac arrhythmia as well as whether the patient has a history of structural heart disease, especially previous myocardial infarction. Also important is whether the patient is taking any medicines, and whether the patient has a pacemaker or internal cardiac defibrillator in place. Initial studies should include an electrocardiogram (ECG) and laboratory values, including serum potassium, magnesium, and cardiac enzymes.

Analysis of the 12 lead ECG is critical to determine the etiology of the arrhythmia. Assessment of the ECG includes evaluation of the regularity of the rhythm, the atrial rate, the P wave morphology, and the relationship between atrial and ventricular rates. Sinus tachycardia is characterized by a 1:1 relationship between atrial and ventricular rates with normal P waves and a heart rate between 100 and 180 beats/min. Atrial tachycardia is characterized by an atrial rate of 100–250 beats/min, but with abnormal P wave morphology and long PR intervals. Atrial flutter has an atrial rate usually of 300 beats/min and a ventricular rate one half to one third the atrial rate. Atrial flutter will present classically with a regular ventricular rate of 150 beats/min (2-to-1 block), but may vary between 3-to-1 and 4-to-1 block (regular heart rates of 100 and 75 beats/min). In contrast, atrial fibrillation (Fig. 4.1) is characterized by a lack of organized atrial activity, with no clear P waves between QRS complexes, and a irregular ventricular response.

Wide complex tachycardia is most often ventricular tachycardia (VT) (Fig. 4.2). The most common algorithm for the diagnosis of wide complex tachycardia is the Brugada criteria, which consists of four steps. The first step is to evaluate for absence of an RS complex in all precordial leads (V1–V6), which is diagnostic of VT with 100% specificity. If an RS complex is present, the RS interval is measured; if the interval is greater than 100 ms, then VT can be diagnosed with 98% specificity. The third step involves looking for evidence of AV dissociation of less than 100 ms in the RS interval, which has a high specificity but a low sensitivity. The final step involves consideration of the morphology of the QRS complex, which has a lower specificity and sensitivity. Torsades de pointes is a polymorphic VT with variability in both the amplitude and

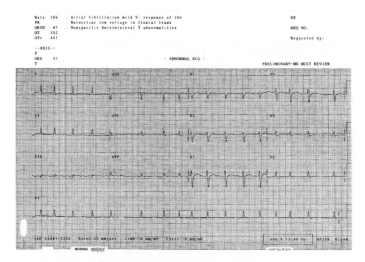

FIGURE 4.1. ECG demonstrating atrial fibrillation.

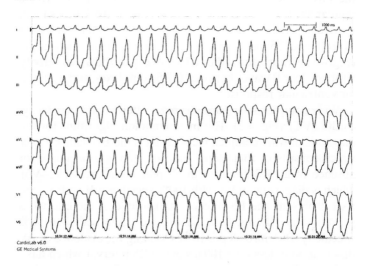

FIGURE 4.2. ECG demonstrating ventricular tachycardia.

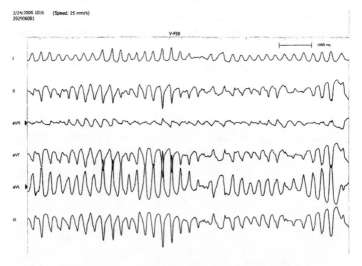

FIGURE 4.3. ECG demonstrating ventricular fibrillation.

polarity, causing the complexes to appear as if they are twisting around the isoelectric line. A prerequisite for the development of Torsades is prolongation of the QT interval. The ECG in ventricular fibrillation (Fig. 4.3) shows complexes that are grossly irregular without P waves or clear QRS morphology.

Treatment

Narrow Complex Arrhythmias

The underlying cause of the arrhythmia should be sought and reversed at the onset if possible. A hemodynamically unstable patient or a patient with acute angina with a narrow complex tachyarrhythmia should be treated expeditiously with DC cardioversion. In the clinically and hemodynamically stable patient, an attempt should be made to determine the rhythm. Sinus tachycardia is the most common tachycardia and is managed by treating the underlying disorder. Atrial flutter, an inherently unstable rhythm, will usually convert acutely to either normal sinus rhythm or to atrial fibrillation. In a stable patient with atrial flutter, control of the ventricular response rate can be achieved with calcium channel blocker, beta blockers, or digoxin. Narrow complex supraventricular tachycardia can be treated with vagal maneuvers, adenosine, or rate control with beta blockade or calcium channel blockers.

The management of atrial fibrillation (Fig. 4.4) is based on the hemodynamic stability of the patient. If the patient is hemodynamically unstable, direct current (DC) cardioversion is the treatment option of choice to restore sinus rhythm. In the hemodynamically stable patient, acute treatment strategies include rate control, termination of the atrial fibrillation with maintenance of sinus rhythm, and antiembolic therapy, depending on whether there is a history of atrial fibrillation in the patient. If atrial fibrillation has been present for more than 48 h, appropriate anticoagulation should be started prior to medical or electrical cardioversion due to the risk of embolic disease from clot in the atrium. Early cardioversion may be considered after appropriate intravenous heparinization and transesophageal echocardiography to rule out atrial thrombus. After cardioversion, management should be followed by

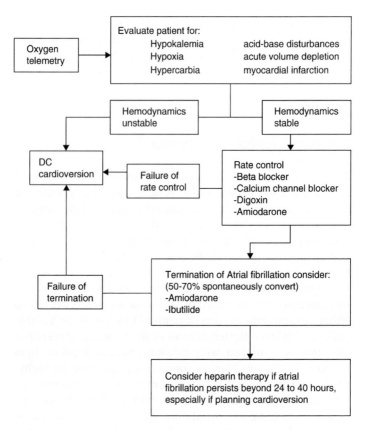

FIGURE 4.4. Algorithm for the management of atrial fibrillation.

4 weeks of anticoagulation. If clot is present, delayed cardioversion may be performed after several weeks of anticoagulation therapy, which again should be continued for a period of weeks after the cardioversion.

Spontaneous conversion rates are as high as 50–70% in the first 24 h after the onset of atrial fibrillation. Beta blockers and calcium channel blockers used to control the ventricular response rate in atrial fibrillation rarely will terminate the rhythm. Digoxin is used as an add-on to either calcium channel blockers or beta blockers to control the ventricular rate and is a good choice in the patient with decompensated heart failure because of the positive inotropic effect. Ibutilide is an antiarrhythmic agent that has efficacy in terminating recent onset atrial fibrillation and atrial flutter[3] and also increases the success rate for electrical conversion. Amiodarone is useful to prolong the AV refractoriness and slow the ventricular response, with a conversion rate of 60%, similar to placebo at 24 h. Because of its long half-life, oral amiodarone leads to effective prolongation of atrial refractoriness and is useful for medical cardioversion; 25% of patients with persistent atrial fibrillation convert to sinus rhythm within 4–6 weeks. Electrical DC cardioversion is another option for conversion to a sinus rhythm, with care taken to anticoagulate the patient appropriately who has been in atrial fibrillation for longer than 48 h to decrease the risk of emboli.

Wide Complex Arrhythmias

Asymptomatic, premature ventricular contractions are common and do not require treatment. No medical therapy is indicated for patients with asymptomatic, hemodynamically stable, non-sustained VT. Underlying abnormalities, such as electrolyte disturbances, hypoxia, structural heart disease, and acute myocardial ischemia, should be ruled out in the setting of non-sustained VT. Patients with sustained VT or ventricular fibrillation should be treated according to ACLS protocols.

The treatment of stable, monomorphic VT depends on the ventricular function. For patients with preserved ventricular function, cardioversion, amiodarone (150 mg IV bolus over 10 min) or procainamide (17 mg/kg load using 20 mg/min followed by 1–4 mg/min IV drip) are acceptable options. For patients with low ejection fractions, amiodarone (150 mg IV bolus) is the treatment of choice. Lidocaine is now considered a secondary agent, because it has limited effect in non-ischemic tissue.

The management of stable, polymorphic VT depends on the duration of the QT interval. Cardioversion is recommended for polymorphic VT with a normal QT interval, because this rhythm is associated often with instability. Electrolyte abnormalities should be corrected, and evidence of ischemia should be sought and treated. Medical therapy for polymorphic VT with normal QT interval includes amiodarone, procainamide, and lidocaine as a secondary agent. Treatment for polymorphic VT with a prolonged QT interval (Torsades) includes IV magnesium and correction of all electrolyte abnormalities. Temporary pacing or IV isoproterenol increases the underlying heart rate and shortens the QT interval, which halts the torsades.

Unstable patients with wide complex tachycardia of any type should be cardioverted. Patients with unstable VT and ventricular fibrillation (VF) are treated with acute cardioversion. If a defibrillator is not immediately available, a precordial thump can be performed immediately after demonstrating pulselessness. Shock is administered first as 200 J, followed by 300 J, then 360 J. If the patient has persistent VT/VF, either epinephrine (1 mg IV) or vasopressin (40 units IV) are given. Amiodarone (300 mg IV) should be given if the patient fails to cardiovert after three rounds of defibrillation.

Selected Readings

Brugada P, Brugada J, Mont L, et al. (1991) A new approach to the differential diagnosis of a regular tachycardia with a wide QRS complex. Circulation 83:1649–1659

Cummins RO (2004) ACLS provider manual, 3rd edn. American Heart Association, Dallas, TX

Naccerelli G, Wolbrette D, Khan M, et al. (2003) Old and new antiarrhythmic drugs for converting and maintaining sinus rhythm in atrial fibrillation: comparative efficacy and results of trials. Am J Cardiol 91:15D–26D

Polanczyc C, Goldman L, Marcantonio E, et al. (1998) Supraventricular arrhythmia in patients having noncardiac surgery. Ann Int Med 129:279–285

Tielman R, Gosselink A, Crijns H, et al. (1997) Efficacy, safety, and determinants of conversion of atrial fibrillation and flutter with oral amiodarone. Am J Cardiol 79:1054–1059

5
Do Not Resuscitate, Do Not Treat

Laurence B. McCullough and James W. Jones

Pearls and Pitfalls

- Ethics represents an essential component of the modern practice of surgery.
- The tools of ethics include the analysis of concepts and the use of concepts to establish measures regarding surgical management and diagnosis.
- "Do-not-Resuscitate" orders should be negotiated with patients, or the surrogates of patients who cannot participate in decision-making of the informed consent process.
- The living will or directive to physicians is an advance directive that patients use to instruct physicians about the administration of life-sustaining treatment when the patient becomes terminally ill and has lost decision-making capacity.
- A directive to physicians serves as the basis for DNR orders for terminally ill patients who cannot participate in decision making, because such an advance directive provides documentation of the patient's decision about the administration of life-sustaining treatment.
- A Durable Power of Attorney for Health Care or Medical Power of Attorney is a written advance directive by which a patient appoints someone to act as the patient's surrogate decision maker when the patient has lost decision-making capacity.

K.I. Bland et al. (eds.), *Critical Care Surgery*,
DOI 10.1007/978-1-84996-378-7_5,
© Springer-Verlag London Limited 2011

- It is ethically justified for DNR orders to be suspended in the OR for patients with terminal conditions and may be re-instated when clinical judgment supports the view that life-threatening events will be owed to the patient's underlying terminal condition rather than anesthesia, surgery, and their side-effects.
- A DNR order does not imply that the patient should not be treated. Appropriate pain management, maintenance of dignity, and assuring the comfort of patients who will be allowed to die is ethically required.

Introduction

Ethics is an essential component of the modern practice of surgery. Ethics uses two tools, analysis of concepts and arguments that use these concepts to reach reasoned conclusions, to guide surgeons in making judgments about beliefs and behaviors. Surgeons are familiar with the clinical utility of ethics, inasmuch as it shapes the informed consent process between surgeons and patients about the surgical management of patients' diseases and injuries. It is worth noting that surgeons pioneered the practice of informed consent, starting with simple consent for surgery in seventeenth-century England leading to a sophisticated form of informed consent already in the nineteenth-century United States, well before the development of the doctrine of informed consent in the common and statutory law in the United States and other countries during the twentieth century. DNR orders are based on informed consent. They formalize agreement between physician and patient/surrogates assuring that resuscitation will be limited at critical junctures in a patient's illness.

History of ethical debate about DNR in the OR

Challenging ethical issues arise in the clinical management of patients with serious illness, i.e., diagnoses with a high probability of death even with aggressive clinical intervention.

Especially challenging is the place of do-not-resuscitate (DNR) orders in the operating room for patients with advance directives. Advance directives are legal instruments through which a patient makes decisions about life-sustaining treatment that are to be respected and implemented when the patient is, in the attending physician's clinical judgment, no longer able to make decisions for himself or herself. The living will or directive to physicians is used to instruct physicians about the administration or withholding of life-sustaining treatment when the patient has lost decision-making capacity and has a terminal condition (as defined in applicable statutory law). The durable power of attorney for health care or the medical power of attorney is used to appoint someone of the patient's choice, known as an agent or proxy, to make decisions for the patient when the patient is no longer able to do so. Either through a directive to physicians or through a medical power of attorney, a surgeon may be validly instructed in advance by a patient with a terminal condition that he or she does not want life-sustaining treatment administered, including resuscitation. Nevertheless, it is sometimes the case that a terminally ill patient can benefit clinically from surgical management of his or her condition or problem.

When this issue first surfaced about 15 years ago, some argued that DNR orders should be applicable in the operating room as they are anywhere else in the hospital. The argument in support of this position appeals to the ethical principle of respect for autonomy. This principle was understood to mean that the informed preferences of patients regarding end of life care should guide physicians' clinical judgment, decision making, and behavior in all clinical settings. Otherwise, advance directives would have little force or meaning if surgeons could simply override directives at the surgeon's discretion.

Others argued that DNR orders should be suspended in all cases when a patient was taken to surgery. Anesthesiologists and surgeons quite reasonably took the view that intraoperative arrest of a seriously or terminally ill patients should be regarded as a correctable side-effect of anesthesia and not a function of the patient's underlying disease or injury. Moreover, intraoperative resuscitation maintains homeostasis and patients usually recover, in sharp contrast to the overall all low success rate of resuscitation elsewhere in the hospital. It seems inconsistent with professional integrity of surgical clinical judgment and practice to withhold intervention that is effective in achieving the goals of surgery. Seriously or terminally ill patients who consent to surgery can reasonable be presumed to want its functional improvements and palliative effects, but they will not experience these outcomes if an intervention that is usually effective in helping to achieve them is withheld. In short, a strong case can be made on both clinical grounds and on the basis of a reasonable assumption about patients' preferences that DNR orders should be suspended during surgery for seriously ill or terminally ill patients.

Critical assessment of positions on DNR in the OR

When these two positions and the arguments in support of them are subjected to close scrutiny, a major problem with the autonomy-based approach, i.e., routinely implementing DNR orders in the OR, suffers from a serious misconception of the role of the patient's autonomy in the ethics of informed consent and, by extension, advance directives. The first step of the informed consent process is for the surgeon to identify the medically reasonable alternatives for managing the patient's condition or problem, i.e., those that are reliably expected to result in a greater balance of clinical goods over harms for the patient. For patients who are otherwise expected to survive a surgical procedure, death cannot be reasonably construed as a benefit. Thus, continuing DNR status intraoperatively is not medically reasonable. This conclusion is buttressed by the consideration above that maintaining DNR status in the OR is not consistent with professional integrity. If the patient preferred the benefits of an earlier timing of death from a terminal condition, then the patient should refuse surgery, including palliative surgery. The patient, however, does not get to define what is medically reasonable or to require surgeons to act in ways that are not consistent with professional integrity.

Ethical consensus concerning DNR in the OR

There has emerged a consensus that it is ethically justified for DNR orders to be suspended in the OR for patients with terminal conditions, including patients who have completed an advance directive that refuses life-sustaining treatment. It is not enough, however, to take the view that DNR orders should be suspended in the OR, because this position does not address the important ethical question of when DNR should be re-instated post operatively. There has emerged a consensus view that DNR status should be restored when life-threatening events are reliably judged to be owed to the patient's underlying terminal condition rather than to anesthesia, surgery, and their side-effects.

What is not mentioned is the fact that although active treatment of problems, from an anesthetic or a procedure, is similar to cardiopulmonary resuscitation, they almost always precede full-blown cardio-pulmonary arrest. As such they are therapies to reverse arrhythmias, hypotension, or hypoxia before the conditions result in cardiopulmonary arrest.

Surgeons should take a preventive ethics approach to DNR in the OR, by talking frankly with patients who remain able to make decisions, or their surrogate decision maker, for patients who do not about the role of DNR in patient care and why DNR status is not medically reasonable intraoperatively. A clear plan should be presented for the timing of a discussion about the re-instatement of DNR status and the surgeon should adhere to this plan. This preventive ethics approach protects both professional integrity and the autonomy of the patient, either as directly exercised by the patient or as indirectly exercised by the patient's surrogate decision maker.

DNR Does Not Mean Do Not Treat

Surgical management of the clinical problems of seriously or terminally ill patients has become an important component of effective palliative care for such patients. Surgeons should keep this larger context in mind, because it helps them to focus on the overall goal of providing appropriate clinical care for terminally ill patients, especially in their last days and hours. Surgeons have a heavily vested interest in providing definitive therapy; as a major part of the surgical persona and the modern armamentarium available emphasizes that role. Hospital mortality rates of individual surgeons are figured into many databases for various purposes. But aside from these distractions, there are many times where relief of bowel obstruction, a tracheotomy, stabilization of a fracture, placement of a supra-pubic cystostomy tube, or the like may bring comfort from torment, which is after all the foundational purpose of medicine.

Selected Readings

Faden RR, Beauchamp TL (1986) A history and theory of informed consent. Oxford University Press, New York

Halevy A, Baldwin JC (1998) Poor surgical risk patients. In: McCullough LB, Jones JW, Brody BA (eds) Surgical ethics. Oxford University Press, New York, pp 152–170

McCullough LB, Jones JW, Brody BA (eds) (1998) Surgical ethics. Oxford University Press, New York

McCullough LB, Jones JW, Brody BA (1998) Informed consent: autonomous decision making and the surgical patient. In: McCullough LB, Jones JW, Brody BA (eds) Surgical ethics. Oxford University Press, New York, pp 15–37

McCullough LB, Coverdale JH, Chervenak FA (2004) Argument-based ethics: a formal tool for critically appraising the normative medical ethics literature. Am J Obstet Gynecol 191:1097–1102

Powderly KE (2000) Patient consent and negotiation in the Brooklyn gynecological practice of Alexander J.C. Skene: 1863–1900. J Med Philos 25:12–27

Walter RM (1991) DNR in the OR: resuscitation as an operative risk. JAMA 266:2407–2412

Wear A (1993) Medical ethics in early modern England. In: Wear A, Geyer-Kordesch J, French R (eds) Doctors and ethics: the earlier historical setting of professional ethics. Rodopi, Amsterdam, The Netherlands, pp 98–130

Wear S, Milch R, Weaver LW (1998) Care of dying patients. In: McCullough LB, Jones JW, Brody BA (eds) Surgical ethics. Oxford University Press, New York, pp 171–197

Youngner SJ, Shuck JM (1998) Advance directives and the determination of death. In McCullough LB, Jones JW, Brody BA (eds) Surgical ethics. Oxford University Press, New York, pp 57–77

6

Multiple Organ Dysfunction: The Systemic Host Response to Critical Surgical Illness

John C. Marshall

Pearls and Pitfalls

- Fluid resuscitation and hemodynamic stabilization is the first priority in the management of a patient with sepsis or SIRS.
- Resuscitation can be expedited and optimized through the use of a resuscitation algorithm.
- Adequate volume resuscitation may compromise respiratory function, and necessitate intubation and mechanical ventilation.
- SIRS is a symptom complex, not a diagnosis and many, but not all, patients may have underlying infection as the cause.
- A presumptive source and bacteriologic diagnosis of infection should be established, and appropriate broad spectrum systemic antibiotics administered.
- Antibiotics should be discontinued within 3 days if no infection is identified, and be only rarely given for a period longer than 7 days.
- A focus of infection amenable to source control measures should be sought, and appropriate interventions performed.
- Patients with significant organ dysfunction should be managed in an intensive care unit (ICU).
- Optimal ICU management requires full attention to the potential harm resulting from critical care interventions.

K.I. Bland et al. (eds.), *Critical Care Surgery*,
DOI 10.1007/978-1-84996-377-7_6,
© Springer-Verlag London Limited 2011

- The Multiple Organ Dysfunction Syndrome is the outcome of systemic homeostatic changes of SIRS, and the de novo injury associated with ICU intervention.

Introduction

The Multiple Organ Dysfunction Syndrome or MODS is the leading cause of death for critically ill patients admitted to an intensive care unit. This snippet of epidemiologic data — intuitively evident to any clinician who has taken care of the multiply injured, hemodynamically unstable, or overwhelmingly infected patient — belies an intimidating complex mélange of pathologic insights that have emerged in parallel with our capacity to sustain the lives of patients who previously would have died of natural causes. Organ dysfunction, and the intimidating complex innate immune mechanisms that give rise to it, have only emerged as important mechanisms of disease as modern medicine has acquired the capacity to treat entities such as shock and infection, which in an earlier era, were rapidly lethal. Moreover, the injury complex that characterizes MODS is an amalgam created not only by the initial life-threatening insult, but even more importantly by the innate host response to that insult, and by the consequences of the therapeutic interventions that the clinician uses to sustain vital organ dysfunction. MODS is the quintessential iatrogenic disorder; it arises because modern medicine is capable of subverting previously lethal processes, but evolves as a direct consequence of the interventions used to sustain life.

The Acute Response to Danger: An Overview

Complex organisms — humans included — have evolved multiple, frequently overlapping mechanisms to respond to threats that pose a risk to life and limb. Blood, for example, is a liquid suspension that circulates under pressure within the vascular tree. In the absence of the coagulation cascade, the most trivial injury would result in exsanguinations and death. However, uncontrolled coagulation also poses a threat, since it arrests blood flow, and so prevents oxygen delivery to tissues. The complexities of normal coagulation and fibrinolysis reflect the twin biologic imperatives of adequately responding to the danger of bleeding, while minimizing the attendant harm of coagulation.

If the biology of the coagulation cascade is discouragingly complex, that of the innate immune response to infection or other external threats is many magnitudes more so. Indeed coagulation and anti-coagulation comprise part of a larger network of innate host defenses, for it is activation of the coagulation cascade and deposition of fibrin that creates an abscess, and activation of anticoagulant mechanisms that permit its resolution.

A comprehensive discussion of the biology of inflammation is far beyond the scope of this chapter. In general terms, it involves multiple biochemical cascades, each with its own counter-regulatory mechanisms that are activated when cells of the host innate immune system perceive danger. For example, activation of the coagulation cascade by microbial products results in the engagement of complement receptors on neutrophils, priming them for amplified production of reactive oxygen species in response to conserved microbial products. It is instructive, however, to review one of the most important of these — the toll-like receptor pathway — for insights it provides into the clinical expression of sepsis.

Toll-like Receptors (TLR) and the Innate Host Response to Danger

Cells of the innate immune system — monocytes, macrophages, and neutrophils in particular — are genetically programmed to recognize danger, and so can respond rapidly, but non-specifically, to a broad spectrum of potentially lethal threats in the local environment. These threats may be invading micro-organisms such as bacteria, fungi, or viruses, but might equally be products released from injured or dying cells in the local environment. Remarkably, this capacity rests with the ability of a family of ten proteins expressed on the surface of these cells to bind, and respond to a broad array of such signals. These cellular receptors are called toll-like receptors or TLRs — not because they extract a toll, but because they are remarkably similar to a very intriguing protein found in the fruit fly that determines which aspect of the fly is the front and which the back. All in all, that role is quite cool, and "toll" is German for "cool."

TLR4, for example, is the receptor that recognizes and binds endotoxin or lipopolysaccharide — a major component of the cell wall of all Gram-negative bacteria. When TLR4 binds endotoxin, a cascade of intracellular events is activated, that ultimately leads to altered expression of no fewer than 3,147 genes in humans — roughly an eighth of all the genes in the entire human genome (Fig. 6.1). Multiple intracellular proteins participate in the intracellular cascade that evokes this genetic response, and so are potentially attractive targets for therapy in the future. But for our purposes, it is sufficient to appreciate that the immediate response to TLR engagement is increased production of key early protein mediators or cytokines, predominant amongst which are tumor necrosis factor (TNF) and interleukin-1 (IL-1). These mediators, in turn, activate other cells, triggering the changes in capillary permeability, vascular reactivity, and intravascular coagulation that result in the clinical picture of sepsis. For example, cytokine-induced increased activity of inducible nitric oxide synthase results in increased generation of nitric oxide, a potent vasodilator that is responsible for the diffuse vasodilatation that is characteristic of resuscitated sepsis. Cytokine-induced increases in the expression of tissue factor on endothelial cells triggers intravascular activation of the coagulation cascade, while the cytokine interleukin-6 triggers the altered pattern of liver protein synthesis that is known as the acute phase response.

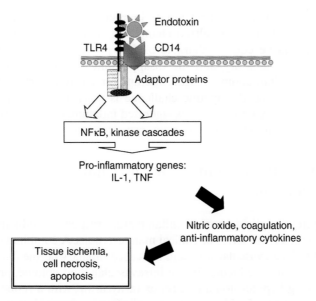

FIGURE 6.1. Schematic representation of the cellular response to danger. Endotoxin from the cell wall of Gram-negative bacteria binds to a cell surface receptor, TLR4, resulting in the aggregation of a number of adapter proteins that associate with the intracellular tail of the receptor. This process initiates an enzymatic cascade, mediated through the addition or removal of phosphate groups from intracellular proteins. Enzymes that add phosphate groups are called kinases, whereas those that remove them are known as phosphatases. The process promotes the passage of transcription factors such as NFκB to the nucleus; these transcription factors bind to DNA, promoting its transcription to RNA, which in turn leads to the synthesis of new proteins. The initial response results in the synthesis of early inflammatory cytokines such as TNF and IL-1; these, in turn, can act on the cell to induce the expression of a large number of genes involved in the acute response to danger. For example, expression of tissue factor initiates the coagulation cascade, while upregulation of inducible nitric oxide synthase leads to the generation of nitric oxide, a potent vasodilator. The consequences of these processes is intravascular thrombosis, maldistribution of tissue blood flow, and cell death, through necrosis or apoptosis, and hence the clinical presentation of organ dysfunction.

The activation of an innate immune response results in profound and generalized changes in systemic homeostasis that can be equally characterized as pro-inflammatory and anti-inflammatory, and the disappointing results of clinical trials of immunomodulatory therapy for sepsis underline the fact that the therapeutic challenge is much more complex than simply blunting an exaggerated inflammatory response, or augmenting a state of immunosuppression.

Systemic Inflammation: The Clinical Syndrome

Systemic activation of an inflammatory response results in a characteristic series of clinical manifestations. A combination of reduced vascular tone and increased capillary permeability results in a reduction in the intravascular fluid volume, producing hypotension and a reflex tachycardia, with a reduced urine output. Fluid resuscitation will often correct the hypotension, but increased capillary permeability leads to interstitial edema; this edema in the lung leads to tachypnea and hypoxia. Confusion presents - as a result of multiple factors including the altered metabolic state, hypoxia, and cerebral edema. The core temperature is typically increased, but may be low; laboratory manifestations reflect a state of systemic inflammation with leukocytosis (or leucopenia in the early stages), hyperglycemia, and evidence of the activation of an acute phase response (hypoalbuminemia and increased levels of C-reactive protein). Several other manifestations of altered organ function may also be present. Indeed, the clinical syndrome is the systemic equivalent of the cardinal manifestations of local inflammation described by Galen and Celsus 2,000 years ago: rubor (vasodilatation), calor (fever), tumor (increased capillary permeability with edema), dolor (malaise and confusion), and functio laesa (organ dysfunction).

While clinical features may vary from one patient to the next, the resultant syndrome is known as the Systemic Inflammatory Response Syndrome (SIRS) (Table 6.1). When

TABLE 6.1. Terminology and definitions.

SIRS

A clinical syndrome resulting from the disseminated activation of an acute inflammatory response, and characterized by two or more of:

Tachycardia (heart rate >90 beats/min)

Tachypnea (respiratory rate >20 breaths/min, PaCO$_2$ <32 mmHg or mechanical ventilation)

Hyper-or hypothermia (temperature >38°C or <36°C)

Leukocytosis or leukopenia (white cell count >11,000 cells/mm^3 or <4,000 cells/mm^3, or >10% band forms)

Infection

The presence of micro-organisms invading normally sterile host tissues

Sepsis

The systemic host response to invasive infection

Severe sepsis

Sepsis in association with organ dysfunction

Septic shock

Sepsis in association with refractory hypotension despite adequate fluid resuscitation

invasive infection is the cause of SIRS, sepsis is present; however SIRS may be present in the absence of infection, and, equally, infection present in the absence of SIRS (Fig. 6.2). The syndrome reflects a spectrum of severity. Severe sepsis is sepsis in association with organ dysfunction, while septic shock is present when the process is of sufficient gravity that cardiovascular collapse is present. Increasing severity is associated with increased risk of mortality; the mortality of septic shock is typically 35–40% or higher.

The mortality risk of sepsis arises both from the presence of uncontrolled infection, and from the consequences of the host response to that infection. In fact the host response, rather than the infection that elicited it, is the most important determinant of survival (Fig. 6.3).

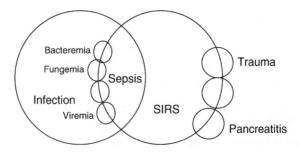

FIGURE 6.2. The relationship between invasive infection and the host response to that process. Note that infection may exist without significant systemic manifestations, and conversely, that a syndrome of systemic inflammation may arise in the absence of infection. When SIRS results from infection, sepsis is said to be present (Data from Bone et al., 1992).

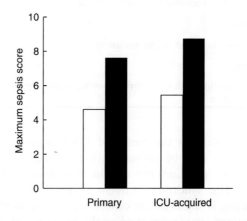

FIGURE 6.3. The severity of the host response, rather than the stimulus that initiated it, is the primary determinant of outcome in critical illness. In a study of 211 critically ill surgical patients, we found that when patients were stratified by infectious status (either primary infection, or infection acquired within the ICU), non-survivors had significantly higher sepsis scores than survivors, indicating a greater degree of clinical response. On the other hand, when patients with elevated sepsis scores were evaluated, no infection-related variables could be found that discriminated survivors from non-survivors (Data from Marshall and Sweeney, 1990).

MODS

The homeostatic changes associated with systemic inflammation can evoke alterations in the function of virtually every organ system. However, six systems predominate: the respiratory, cardiovascular, hematological, gastrointestinal, renal, and central nervous systems. Respiratory dysfunction is also commonly described as the Acute Respiratory Distress Syndrome (ARDS). MODS can be defined as the development of acute and potentially reversible derangements in the function of two or more organ systems. The mortality risk increases with both the number of failing organ systems and the severity of dysfunction within each system, giving rise to a number of scoring systems such as the Multiple Organ Dysfunction (MOD) and the Sequential Organ Failure Assessment (SOFA) scores (Table 6.2).

MODS is a complex process, reflecting both the physiologic consequences of systemic inflammation, and further injury resulting from interventions used to sustain life. For example, overdistention of the lung during mechanical ventilation can exacerbate acute lung injury, and transfusion and a variety of medications can induce renal and hepatic dysfunction. By promoting the emergence of resistant organ¬isms, systemic antibiotics can increase the risk of nosocomial infection and further organ dysfunction. MODS is a fundamentally iatrogenic disorder: it only arises because the clinician has intervened in an otherwise lethal process, but those interventions themselves can cause further injury.

Clinical Management of the Septic Patient

The development of SIRS or sepsis in the surgical patient is a potentially life-threatening situation, and urgent and appropriate intervention is essential to minimize the mortality risk.

The initial priority is resuscitation and hemodynamic support. Fluid resuscitation can be accomplished with either

TABLE 6.2. The Multiple Organ Dysfunction (MOD) score.

Organ system	0	1	2	3	4
Respiratory[a]					
(PO$_2$/FIO$_2$ ratio)	>300	226–300	151–225	76–150	≤75
Renal[b]					
(Serum creatinine)	≤100	101–200	201–350	351–500	>500
Hepatic[c]					
(Serum bilirubin)	≤20	21–60	61–120	121–240	>240
Cardiovascular[d]					
(Pressure-adjusted Heart rate – PAR)	≤10	10.1–15	15.1–20	20.1–30	>30
Hematologic[e]					
(Platelet count)	>120	81–120	51–80	21–50	≤20
Neurologic[f]					
(Glasgow coma score)	15	13–14	10–12	7–9	≤6

[a]The PO2/FIO$_2$ ratio is calculated without reference to the use or mode of mechanical ventilation, and without reference to the use or level of PEEP.
[b]The serum creatinine level is measured in mmol/l, without reference to the use of dialysis.
[c]The serum bilirubin level is measured in mmol/l.
[d]The pressure-adjusted heart rate (PAR) is calculated as the product of the heart rate and right atrial (central venous) pressure, divided by the mean arterial pressure: PAR = Heart rate × CVP divided by MAP.
[e]The platelet count is measured in platelets/ml 10–3.
[f]The glasgow coma score is preferably calculated by the patient's nurse, and is scored conservatively (for the patient receiving sedation or muscle relaxants, normal function is assumed unless there is evidence of intrinsically altered mentation).

sodium-containing crystalloids such as normal saline or Ringer's lactate, or with colloids such as albumin; there are no convincing data to support the superiority of one over the other, and as the cheaper option, crystalloids are often the resuscitative fluid of choice. Effective volume losses may be substantial. The patient should receive an initial bolus infusion of 500 ml to a liter of fluid, followed by additional boluses as needed to raise the blood pressure, reduce the heart rate, and restore urine output to more than 30 ml/h. Often many liters of fluid will be required to accomplish these objectives. Optimal resuscitation can be further facilitated by the insertion of a central venous catheter to permit monitoring of central venous pressure and oxygen saturation ($ScVO_2$). A central venous pressure of at least 8 cm H_2O should be targeted, although often higher levels are needed to improve heart rate and blood pressure. An $ScVO_2$ of 70 or more should be targeted. When the blood pressure fails to respond to volume challenge (a CVP of more than 8) alone, a vasopressor such as norepinephrine should be added. Similarly, an inotropic agent such as dobutamine, or transfusion of packed red cells, should be considered if the $ScVO_2$ fails to respond to volume challenge alone. Used at the time of initial presentation, this resuscitative algorithm — termed goal-directed resuscitation — has been shown to increase the survival of patients with severe sepsis by as much as 16% (Fig. 6.4).

Cultures of blood and other potential infectious foci should be drawn as part of the initial phases of resuscitation, followed by administration of systemic broad spectrum

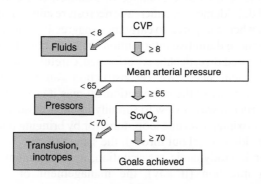

FIGURE 6.4. Goal-directed resuscitation of the patient with septic shock. Intravenous fluid is first administered to increase the CVP to 8 cm H_2O or higher. If this fails to raise the mean arterial pressure to at least 65 mmHg, vasopressors are added, and if the oxygen saturation of blood drawn from the superior vena cava ($ScVO_2$) through the central line is less than 70%, inotropes and blood transfusion are administered (Data from Rivers et al., 2001).

empiric antibiotics — selected on the basis of the presumptive site of infection, and of knowledge of local patterns of bacterial resistance. Comprehensive broad spectrum therapy is provided until culture and sensitivity data are available. The antibiotic spectrum should be narrowed on the basis of these data, and if cultures are negative after 72 h, antibiotics should be discontinued unless there are compelling reasons to suspect undiagnosed infection.

An inciting focus of infection should be sought for each patient with clinical manifestations of sepsis, and once a focus has been identified, appropriate source control measures should be undertaken. Source control interventions can be broadly classified as drainage, debridement and device removal, and definitive management. The need for source control can usually be established on the basis of the clinical presentation, augmented by the findings of radiological examinations such as computed tomography or ultrasonography. As a general principle, the best source control measure is one that accomplishes the source control objective, with the minimal physiologic upset to the patient. Thus percutaneous drainage is preferable to operative drainage of localized collections, and delayed debridement of pancreatic necrosis results in improved survival when compared to early, more aggressive intervention. When a more definitive intervention such as a bowel resection for perforated diverticulitis is performed, careful consideration of subsequent needs for reconstruction can minimize the global morbidity of the intervention. Stomas, if created, should be constructed with a view to simplifying their closure, by creating a proximal diverting loop stoma, or by bringing both ends of the divided bowel out through the same orifice.

After hemodynamic resuscitation, and treatment of the inciting infection (if any), the management of systemic inflammatory response syndrome is supportive — the goal being to support failing vital organ function while minimizing the inevitable harm associated with life support. The goal of mechanical ventilation, for example, is to ensure adequate gas exchange in the lungs to permit oxygen delivery to the tissues, but to do so without further exacerbating acute lung injury.

These potentially competing imperatives can be accomplished by careful consideration of the benefits and harms of intervention. Hemodynamic resuscitation of the septic patient often results in respiratory insufficiency because of increased capillary permeability in the lung. Mechanical ventilation with low tidal volumes (6 ml/kg) can minimize the trauma resulting from the ventilator, and the use of positive end-expiratory pressure (PEEP) keeps lung units open to facilitate gas exchange at low tidal volumes. Provided that oxygen delivery is satisfactory, the fraction of inspired oxygen (F_IO_2) delivered by the ventilator can be set at a level adequate to result in oxygen saturation of the arterial blood (SaO_2) to a level of 92–95%. Finally, it is important to remember that the objective is to liberate the patient from the ventilator, and that daily weaning trials can reduce the duration of mechanical ventilation, and so reduce the associated risks.

Nutritional support should be provided, using the enteral route if at all possible. The benefits of formulae supplemented with anti-oxidants or other immunonutrients are unclear. Strict control of blood sugar levels has shown benefit in populations of critically ill surgical patients, though it remains unclear how tight this control should be. Infection prevention is grounded in efforts to remove unneeded invasive devices, to ensure optimal antiseptic care of those that are needed, and to reduce or eliminate unnecessary antibiotic exposure.

An evidence-based overview of the optimal management of the septic patient is beyond the scope of this brief review, but can be found in the guidelines of the Surviving Sepsis Campaign (www.survivingsepsis.org).

Adjuvant Treatments for Sepsis

Evolving insights into the complex biology of the septic response hold the promise of new modes of adjuvant therapy for a process with a mortality of 30% or higher despite adequate conventional management. Currently however, the options, are limited.

Activated protein C (APC or drotrecogin alpha activated) is an endogenous anticoagulant molecule whose levels are significantly reduced during sepsis. In addition to an anticoagulant activity in limiting microvascular thrombosis, APC can bind to cell receptors, reducing levels of inflammatory cytokines and limiting neutrophil activation. In a multicenter randomized trial of drotrecogin alpha in patients with severe sepsis, treatment was associated with a 20% relative improvement in survival, although the effects were seen only in the more severely ill patients. Controversy regarding the identification of the appropriate population of patients to treat, and the substantial cost of the agent, has limited its use in clinical practice. However, it should be considered in the more severely ill patient with sepsis, and in particular, when coagulopathy is a prominent component of the symptom complex.

Pharmacological doses of corticosteroids (50 mg hydrocortisone four times daily) have shown benefit in several small studies of patients with refractory septic shock, and in one larger multicenter French trial of patients with septic shock and non-responsiveness to an ACTH stimulation test. A more recent European trial has failed to replicate this finding, and so the role of adjuvant corticosteroids remains controversial. Given their low cost, and relatively low adverse event rate (they are, however, associated with prolonged neuromuscular weakness following ICU discharge), their use should be considered in patients with septic shock who remain vasopressor-dependent, despite adequate volume resuscitation.

Other therapeutic approaches remain unproven. A few, such as intravenous immunoglobulin, antithrombin, interferon-gamma, or G-CSF – represent commercially available agents that have shown some promise of efficacy in small studies. Others, such as anti-TNF antibodies or the interleukin-1 receptor antagonist, demonstrate efficacy when the results of clinical trials are pooled, but are not commercially available. Presently, the therapeutic benefit is sufficiently small, the appropriate population for therapy sufficiently undefined, and the therapies themselves sufficiently costly, that they must be considered experimental.

Conclusions

MODS is both a clinical syndrome, and a metaphor for a process of care. The syndrome arises through the activation of a systemic host response to a threat to life — infection, injury, ischemia, for example. The physiologic derangements resulting from that process can be corrected by aggressive and timely intervention aimed at rapidly restoring hemodynamic homeostasis. Infection can be treated with antibiotics and surgical source control, and injury can be repaired. Moreover we are on the edge of a new therapeutic approach, based on modulating the complex changes in innate immune function that underlie the clinical syndrome.

On other hand, MODS reflects not only the successes of critical care, but also its limitations. Prolonged support of failing organ system function does not necessarily lead to its reversal and may, indeed, aggravate existing dysfunction, or induce new injury. The line between extraordinary successes of technological medicine, and inappropriate meddling in the natural process of dying is a remarkably fine one.

Selected Readings

Bone RC, Balk RA, Cerra FB, et al. (1992) ACCP/SCCM Consensus Conference. Definitions for sepsis and organ failure and guidelines for the use of innovative therapies in sepsis. Chest 101:1644–1655

Dellinger RP, Carlet JM, Masur H, et al. (2004) Surviving sepsis campaign guidelines for management of severe sepsis and septic shock. Crit Care Med 32:858–873

Levy MM, Fink M, Marshall JC, et al. (2003) 2001 SCCM/ ESICM/ ACCP/ATS/SIS international sepsis definitions conference. Crit Care Med 34:1250–1256

Marshall JC, Sweeney D (1990) Microbial infection and the septic response in critical surgical illness. Arch Surg 125:17–23

Marshall JC (2003) Such stuff as dreams are made on: mediator-targeted therapy in sepsis. Nature Rev Drug Disc 2:391–405

Marshall JC, Cook DJ, Christou NV, et al. (1995) Multiple organ dysfunction score: a reliable descriptor of a complex clinical outcome. Crit Care Med 23:1638–1652

Rivers E, Nguyen B, Havstad S, et al. (2001) Early goal-directed therapy in the treatment of severe sepsis and septic shock. N Engl J Med 345:1368–1377

7
Hepatic Failure

Patrick K. Kim and Clifford S. Deutschman

Pearls and Pitfalls

- Hepatic failure affects nearly every organ system: neurologic, cardiovascular, gastrointestinal, renal, hematologic, endocrine, and immune.
- Although there are many causes of hepatic failure, few have specific treatments.
- The most common causes of death are cerebral edema, sepsis, and multisystem organ failure.
- Liver transplantation is often the only durable therapy.

The liver plays a central role in substrate and toxin metabolism, protein synthesis, and both innate and acquired immunity. This makes hepatic failure in the surgical patient an extraordinary management challenge. Acetaminophen toxicity is the most common etiology of fulminant hepatic failure in the United States and United Kingdom, but a variety of etiologies can cause hepatic failure (Table 7.1). Untreated hepatic failure is highly lethal and, with a few exceptions, much of the current treatment of hepatic failure is supportive. The most common causes of death after liver failure are cerebral edema and sepsis/multisystem organ failure. Survival after hepatic failure depends upon rapid diagnosis, initiation of supportive measures, and prompt evaluation by a liver transplant team. Liver transplantation is often the only curative therapy.

K.I. Bland et al. (eds.), *Critical Care Surgery*,
DOI 10.1007/978-1-84996-378-7_7,
© Springer-Verlag London Limited 2011

TABLE 7.1. Etiologies of hepatic failure.

Drugs and toxins	*Idiosyncratic*
Acetaminophen	Halothane
Amanita phalloides mushroom	Isoniazid
Methyldioxymethamphetamine	Rifampicin
("Ecstasy")	Valproic acid
Herbal remedies	Disulfiram
Carbon tetrachloride	Nonsteroidal antiinflammatory drugs
Yellow phosphorus	
Sulfonamides	*Cardiovascular*
Tetracycline	Right heart failure
	Budd-Chiari syndrome Veno-occlusive disease
Viruses	Shock liver
Hepatitis A virus	
Hepatitis B virus	*Metabolic*
Hepatitis D virus	Acute fatty liver of pregnancy
Hepatitis E virus	Wilson's disease
Herpes simplex virus	
Cytomegalovirus	*Others*
Epstein-Barr virus	Sepsis
Varicella zoster virus	Autoimmune hepatitis
Adenovirus	Hepatic infiltration by malignancy

Pathogenesis and Pathophysiology

While hepatic dysfunction adversely affects nearly every organ system (Fig. 7.1), the primary defect is an intrinsic failure of hepatocellular synthesis. Simply put, liver cells fail to manufacture the essential products that are required for proper function. This leads to most of the organ dysfunction characteristic of

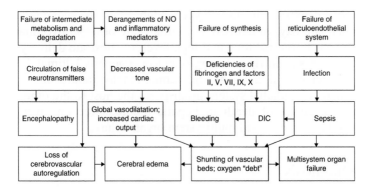

FIGURE 7.1. Pathophysiology of systemic derangements in hepatic failure. NO, nitric oxide; DIC, disseminated intravascular coagulation.

fulminant hepatic failure of chronic cirrhosis. For example, failure to synthesize bile acid and organic anion transporters leads to an inability to clear toxins from the portal and systemic blood. This is reflected in jaundice. Failure to clear byproducts of nitrogen metabolism results in elevations of ammonia and false neurotransmitters. These contribute to encephalopathy, impaired blood-brain barrier and altered cerebrovascular autoregulation. Alterations in hepatic regulation of renal salt handling lead to hyponatremia and total body sodium overload. This may be the basis for the hepato-renal syndrome. The combination of blood-brain barrier dysfunction, hyponatremia and low oncotic pressure from defective albumin synthesis can cause cerebral edema and perhaps coma. Failure of hepatic synthetic function also leads to deficiencies of fibrinogen and coagulation factors II, V, VII, IX, and X. In conjunction with both quantitative and qualitative platelet abnormalities, this results in a profound coagulopathy. The result may be a state of disseminated intravascular coagulation.

Derangements in the metabolism of nitric oxide and inflammatory cytokines cause vasodilatation, hypotension, low systemic vascular resistance and high cardiac output. This hyperdynamic circulation is similar to sepsis. Like sepsis, the combination of metabolic dysfunction and the DIC-induced microvascular thrombosis lead to poor end organ oxygen extraction and oxygen "debt" despite seemingly adequate oxygen delivery. An initial state of hyperglycemia reflects hormonal tone and high levels of substrate delivery, but masks an intrinsic failure of gluconeogenesis. Ultimately, this defect will cause hypoglycemia. Finally, failure of the reticuloendothelial system predisposes the host to the other major causes of death in hepatic failure: infection, overwhelming sepsis, and multisystem organ failure.

Diagnosis

The diagnosis of hepatic failure is based on history, physical examination, and laboratory studies. The symptoms and signs are largely nonspecific and include malaise, fatigue, anorexia, nausea, abdominal pain, fever, and jaundice. The hallmarks of liver failure are encephalopathy, hyperbilirubinemia, and coagulopathy. The severity of each of these predicts poor outcome. Hepatic failure is further classified based on the interval between onset of jaundice and onset of encephalopathy:

Fulminant	<2 weeks
Subfulminant	2 weeks – 3 weeks
Late-onset	8 weeks – 24 weeks

If ascites is present, the serum-to-ascites albumin gradient aids in determining the etiology of ascites (Table 7.2).

TABLE 7.2. Serum-to-ascites albumin gradient (SAAG) and differential diagnosis of etiology of ascites.

SAAG > 1.1	SAAG < 1.1
Cirrhosis	Malignancy
Budd-Chiari syndrome	Pancreatic disease
Cardiac disease	Bile leak
Portal vein thrombosis	Infection
Myxedema	Nephrotic syndrome
Liver metastasis	

Management

Management of the patient begins with assessment of the patient's ability to maintain airway and breathing. Encephalopathy should be characterized (Table 7.3).

Endotracheal intubation and mechanical ventilation should be considered for stages 3 and 4 encephalopathy. As with any patient at risk for life-threatening hemorrhage, the patient should have large-bore intravenous access, preferably peripheral, regardless of whether a central catheter is required for monitoring or for infusion of vasopressors. The blood bank must always have an active type and crossmatch specimen. Serum electrolytes should be monitored frequently for abnormalities of serum sodium and potassium. Blood glucose should be monitored frequently for both hyperglycemia and hypoglycemia. Hematologic and coagulation profiles should be checked serially for trends in hemoglobin/hematocrit, platelet count, prothrombin time, international normalized ratio (INR), and partial thromboplastin time. Liver function tests and serum ammonia are frequently obtained, but contribute little to decision-making in the acute setting.

The intravascular volume should be assessed carefully. Intravascular deficits should be repleted and fluid status reassessed frequently. Fluid resuscitation should start with isotonic solutions. Hypotonic solutions should be avoided, especially with preexisting hyponatremia. Fluid resuscitation should be aggressive in intensity, not necessarily in volume.

TABLE 7.3. West Haven staging of hepatic encephalopathy.

Grade	Description
0	Detectable only by neuropsychological testing
1	Lack of awareness, euphoria or anxiety, shortened attention span, impaired addition or subtraction
2	Lethargy, minimal disorientation to time, personality change, inappropriate behavior
3	Somnolence but responsive to verbal stimuli, confusion, gross disorientation, bizarre behavior
4	Comatose

Fluid overload may lead to complications such as heart failure, pulmonary edema, and abdominal compartment syndrome. Fluid resuscitation should favor colloids such as albumin, given the low oncotic pressure typically encountered. Plasma has the benefit of correcting INR while expanding intravascular volume, but in the patient who is not actively bleeding its routine administration is controversial. Plasma transfusion simply to correct an abnormal INR in the absence of active bleeding is not warranted.

Endpoints of resuscitation should be individualized and chosen carefully. A priori, a reasonable target for mean arterial pressure (MAP) is approximately 65 mmHg, at which point end organ perfusion should be assessed. From an intravascular volume standpoint, central monitoring may be necessary after initial fluid resuscitation, as it is often difficult to clinically gauge intravascular volume status. There are few evidence-based guidelines for the use of central venous pressure or pulmonary artery catheters. The decision to use either catheter remains at the discretion of the treating physician.

The thresholds for transfusion of blood and platelets should be individualized. There are no evidence based guidelines for transfusion triggers in patients with hepatic failure. Given the underlying propensity to hemorrhage, at present it seems prudent to set a transfusion trigger around 8 mg/dl, weighing benefits of transfusion with risks of transfusion reactions, immunosuppression, and predisposition to infection. The classic threshold for platelet transfusion is 50,000/mm^3 if an invasive procedure is being planned and 20,000/mm^3 absolute, at which point spontaneous bleeding may occur. In small studies, recombinant factor VIIa has shown promise in correcting clinical coagulopathy and decreasing transfusion requirement. Further study is warranted.

Diagnosis and treatment of cerebral edema is of paramount importance. Cerebral edema is a life-threatening complication and, if allowed to persist, may exclude the possibility of liver transplantation. Unfortunately, cerebral edema is insidious and diagnosis is clinically difficult. The neurologic exam is usually confounded by encephalopathy or obtundation from medications or other causes. Clinical findings such as decerebrate rigidity, disconjugate gaze, loss of pupillary reflexes, and the Cushing reflex (hypertension with bradycardia) are manifestations of cerebral herniation, a late sequela of cerebral edema, and a grave sign. In the patient with abnormal mental status, computed tomography and magnetic resonance imaging may exclude other diagnoses, but neither modality is sufficiently sensitive to diagnose and quantify cerebral edema. The most accurate (and invasive) method is direct monitoring of intracranial pressure (ICP). The benefits of monitoring of the intracranial pressure must be weighed against the increased risks of bleeding and infection that accompany hepatic failure. Compared to intraparenchymal monitors, extradural monitors have the lowest complication rate and are thus preferred. Intracranial hypertension is present when intracranial pressure is >18–22 mmHg. Cerebral perfusion pressure (CPP) is defined as the difference between mean arterial pressure (MAP) and ICP. Target CPP should be approximately 60 mmHg. The cornerstone of ICP management is mannitol, an osmotic diuretic. The recommended dose range is 0.75–1.25 mg/kg body weight, given every 6–8 h. However, studies in head injury demonstrate that mannitol becomes less effective with each dose and as the total cumulative dose increases. This agent may be administered until serum osmolality reaches 320 mOsmol/kg and/or the osmolar gap (the difference between measures and calculated osmoles) is >55 mOsmol/kg. Hypertonic saline has been shown to decrease ICP in patients with traumatic brain injury, but experience in hepatic cerebral edema is limited and the use of this agent cannot be recommended at this time. Vasopressor therapy should be initiated when hypotension persists, despite correction of hypovolemia or when CPP is impaired. Based on the underlying pathophysiologic derangements, the pressor of choice is norepinephrine. Epinephrine, dobutamine, and dopamine are *not* considered first-line drugs to increase MAP. Hyperventilation, which decreases ICP on the basis of selective cerebral vasoconstriction, is useful acutely. It should not be used persistently because vasoconstriction decreases cerebral blood flow and impairs oxygen delivery. Neither barbiturate nor thiopental coma has proven beneficial in hepatic encephalopathy. Propofol is under investigation. Jugular venous bulb oximetry may provide insight into cerebral oxygen consumption-delivery relationship, but it is unclear from these data whether oximetry improves outcomes. The suggested endpoint is O2 saturation between 65% and 80%. Mild hypothermia has been studied experimentally and is promising. This approach has been shown to decrease ICP by decreasing brain metabolic demand. Studies also suggest that mild hypothermia does not increase bleeding risk. Further study is needed before this therapy can be recommended.

Regarding hepatic encephalopathy, lactulose is the mainstay of therapy. Lactulose acidifies the gut lumen, promoting ammonium ion formation (ammonium ion is not absorbed from the lumen). Lactulose also induces osmotic diarrhea, which removes ammonium from the body. Gut decontamination with metronidazole and oral neomycin theoretically decreases the count of urea-splitting bacteria in the lumen, but it is unclear if this significantly decreases ammonia production. Modified nutritional formulas rich in branched chain and deficient in aromatic amino acids have been studied extensively. They have been shown to improve encephalopathy score, but do not appear to alter outcome.

Bacterial infection occurs in about 80% of patients with hepatic failure, and patients with infection who subsequently develop sepsis are at high-risk for mortality. Although there is debate about which specific regimen is most appropriate, a broad-spectrum antibiotic coverage, most often a 4th generation cephalosporin, probably is warranted. The appropriate duration of prophylactic antibiotic therapy is unclear. Fungal infection occurs in about one-third of patients and similarly portends a poor outcome. At present, it is unclear whether empiric antifungal therapy should be initiated routinely. In patients with suspected infection or sepsis, it is imperative to obtain appropriate cultures immediately, administer broad-spectrum antibiotics, and pursue goal-directed therapy as described for other patients with suspected sepsis.

Renal failure occurs in up to half of patients with hepatic failure and is associated with increased mortality. There is no benefit to infusions of furosemide or dopamine. *Hepatorenal syndrome* is defined as renal dysfunction (serum creatinine >1.5 mg/dl or creatinine clearance < 40 ml/min) with hepatic failure in the absence of prerenal, intrinsic renal, and postrenal etiologies of renal failure (e.g., hypovolemia, shock, nephrotoxin, significant proteinuria, obstructive uropathy). The treatment of renal dysfunction is supportive, with judicious fluid resuscitation and avoidance of nephrotoxic agents. Renal dysfunction may progress to frank renal failure. In such cases, the choice of renal replacement modality depends on hemodynamic stability. In the hemodynamically unstable patient, continuous renal replacement therapy (e.g., continuous venovenous hemodiafiltration) is superior to intermittent hemodialysis in its ability to maintain mean arterial pressure.

Hepatic failure is associated with portal hypertension. Formation of porto-systemic collaterals leads to the development of esophageal varices. Variceal bleeding is a grave sign. Although half of variceal bleeding stops spontaneously, over half of these patients have recurrence within 48 h. Blood and blood products should be rapidly transfused. While at one time vasopressin was the preferred approach to variceal bleeding, this agent has been replaced by octreotide. An octreotide infusion of 250 mcg/h IV × 48 h is as effective as a vasopressin infusion in halting variceal bleeding and is associated with a lower incidence of cardiac and gastrointestinal ischemic complications. Endoscopic band ligation and/or sclerotherapy may be useful. For refractory bleeding, transjugular intrahepatic portosystemic shunt (TIPS) should be considered, with the caveat that the procedure worsens encephalopathy and acutely increases venous return to the heart. Thus, TIPS is relatively contraindicated in patients with pre-existing encephalopathy and cardiac dysfunction. Balloon tamponade may be valuable to consider as a last resort. A variety of balloon tamponade catheters are available. All are based on the same concept: After elective endotracheal intubation and mechanical ventilation, the tube is inserted by the orogastric route. The stomach balloon is inflated and traction is applied to the tube. If bleeding persists, the esophageal balloon is inflated. The balloons are deflated periodically to reduce the risk of pressure necrosis.

TABLE 7.4. Etiologies of hepatic failure with specific treatments.

Etiology of hepatic failure	Treatment
Acetaminophen toxicity	N-acetylcysteine
Herpes simplex hepatitis	Acyclovir
Acute fatty liver of pregnancy	Delivery of fetus
Wilson's disease	Copper chelating agents
Amanita mushroom poisoning	Penicillin and silibinin

As mentioned previously, much of the care is supportive. There are only a few etiologies of hepatic failure with specific therapies (Table 7.4). For many cases of hepatic failure, liver transplantation is the only durable therapy.

Prognosis and Outcome Prediction

The King's College Criteria for Liver Transplantation, initially described in 1980, is widely used for evaluating severity of hepatic failure (Table 7.5). There is significant experience in its application both for acetaminophen and non-acetaminophen etiologies of hepatic failure. The criteria are quite sensitive in patients with acetaminophen toxicity; those patients who fulfill the criteria have poor outcomes. However, the criteria have poor specificity and negative predictive value for both acetaminophen toxicity and non-acetaminophen causes. That is, many patients who do not fulfill the criteria have poor outcomes.

More recently, the Model for End-Stage Liver Disease (MELD) score has been used to stratify degree of hepatic failure. In contrast to the Child-Turcotte-Pugh score (Table 7.6) the MELD score does not incorporate evaluation of ascites and encephalopathy, which are somewhat subjective. Rather, the MELD score is determined solely by three ubiquitous laboratory studies: serum creatinine, serum bilirubin, and INR (Fig. 7.2).

The MELD score, originally developed to predict short-term survival after TIPS procedures, has been validated statistically and has been used since 2002 by the United Network

TABLE 7.5. King's College criteria for liver transplantation.

Acetaminophen toxicity	Non-acetaminophen etiologies
pH < 7.3	PT > 100 s (INR > 6.5)
or **all** of the following	or **any three** of the following
Grade III–IV encephalopathy	Age <10 or >40 Years
PT > 100 s (INR > 6.5)	PT > 50 s (INR > 3.5)
Serum creatinine >3.4 mg/dl	Serum bilirubin >17.5 mg/dl
	Period of jaundice to encephalopathy >7 days
	Etiology is non-A, non-B hepatitis, halothane toxicity, idiosyncratic drug reaction, or Wilson's disease

PT, prothrombin time; INR, international normalized ratio.

TABLE 7.6. Child-Turcotte-Pugh Score.

Criteria	Points 1	2	3
Ascites	None	Slight	Moderate
Bilirubin	≤2	2–3	>3
Albumin	>3.5	2.8–3.5	<2.8
INR	<1.7	1.8–2.3	>2.3
Encephalopathy	None	Grades 1 or 2	Grades 3 or 4

Score	**Grade**	**1-Year survival (%)**	**2-Year survival (%)**
5–6	A	100	85
7–9	B	80	60
10–15	C	45	35

INR, international normalized ratio.

$$R = 9.6 \times \log_e(\text{serum Cr, mg/dL}) + 3.8 \times \log_e(\text{serum bilirubin, mg/dL}) + 11.20 \times \log_e(\text{INR}) + 6.4$$

FIGURE 7.2. Calculation of Model for End-stage Liver Disease (MELD) score. Cr, creatinine; INR, international normalized ratio.

for Organ Sharing (UNOS) for allocation of livers for transplantation. The key to successful transplantation is early evaluation by a dedicated transplant team. If not already in one, the patient should be transferred promptly to a liver transplant center. General contraindications to liver transplantation include extrahepatic malignancy, uncontrolled sepsis, multiple organ failure, and intractable cerebral edema (e.g., sustained ICP >50 mmHg or CPP <40 mmHg).

A variety of short-term alternatives to orthotopic liver transplantation have been proposed. Among the treatments that have been studied are total hepatectomy with portacaval shunting, bioartificial liver, heterotopic liver transplantation, and xenotransplantation. Unfortunately, none has been sufficiently successful to be used clinically.

Conclusion

In summary, hepatic failure is one of the most challenging clinical problems to manage. Nearly every organ system is affected by hepatic failure: neurologic, cardiovascular, gastrointestinal, renal, hematologic, endocrine, and immune. Rapid diagnosis and treatment is essential and early referral to a transplant center is imperative. Cerebral edema, sepsis, and multisystem organ failure are the most common causes of mortality.

Selected Readings

Eghtesad B, Kadry Z, Fung J (2005) Technical considerations in liver transplantation: what a hepatologist needs to know (and every surgeon should practice). Liver Transpl 11:861–871

Jalan R (2003) Intracranial hypertension in acute liver failure: pathophysiological basis of rational management. Semin Liver Dis 23:271–282

Jalan R (2005) Acute liver failure: current management and future prospects. J Hepatol 42:S115–S123

Kamath PS, Wiesner RH, Malinchoc M, et al. (2001) A model to predict survival in patients with end-stage liver disease. Hepatology 33:464–470

O'Grady JG, Alexander GJ, Hayllar KM, Williams R (1989) Early indicators of prognosis in fulminant hepatic failure. Gastroenterology 97:439–445

Sass DA, Shakil AO (2005) Fulminant hepatic failure. Liver Transpl 11:594–605

8
General Principles of Sepsis

Gordon L. Carlson and Paul M. Dark

Pearls and Pitfalls

- Sepsis is a mediator disease, characterized by the host immune and inflammatory response to an infection.
- The outcome of sepsis is critically dependent upon eradicating its source – other aspects of therapy are supportive in nature.
- Prompt recognition and intervention is essential to avoid the development of severe sepsis and septic shock, for which prognosis remains poor.
- Early signs of sepsis in surgical patients may be subtle and easily overlooked and a high degree of suspicion is warranted, especially in the postoperative patient.
- Blood cultures are frequently negative or misleading.
- Radiological management may permit drainage of infected fluid collections, but surgical management is essential in the presence of necrotic tissue and may be the only effective means of establishing adequate source control.

Epidemiology of Sepsis

Infection remains a major cause of morbidity and mortality in general surgical practice, despite advances in perioperative care and refinements in antimicrobial chemotherapy.

K.I. Bland et al. (eds.), *Critical Care Surgery*,
DOI 10.1007/978-1-84996-378-7_8,
© Springer-Verlag London Limited 2011

Ever more complex surgical procedures are being undertaken on an increasingly aged, frail, and comorbid patient population, with specific risk factors for infective complications, including diabetes, malignant disease, and implantation of prosthetic material. Recent estimates in the USA suggest that septic shock accounts for approximately 100,000 deaths each year, is the 13th most common cause of death and, despite the investment of many billions of dollars in novel antimicrobial chemotherapeutic agents, refinements in techniques for organ support, and immunotherapy, there has been little, if any, significant improvement in the outcome of treatment for septic shock for 2 decades. Overall, mortality rates following admission to the intensive care unit (ICU) with septic shock remain approximately 50%. Sepsis syndrome occurs in 400,000 patients per annum in the USA, with surgical patients accounting for almost one third of cases.

Definitions

Sepsis is a disease characterized by the host mediator response to an infection. Many of the clinical and biochemical features that characterize sepsis are related to the release of endogenous mediators, in response to microbial products, including pro-inflammatory cytokines such as tumor necrosis factor alpha and interleukins 1 and 6. Release of these mediators can also be induced, however, by noninfective stimuli, including extensive tissue injury, massive blood transfusion, and sterile inflammation, for example, in acute severe pancreatitis. An international consensus has enabled a logical approach to this spectrum of illness, by recognizing that the clinical consequences of endogenous mediator release comprise the systemic inflammatory response syndrome (SIRS), and that sepsis is defined as the development of SIRS as a consequence of infection (Table 8.1). In addition to these definitions of sepsis, the classification takes into account sepsis severity, including sepsis syndrome (severe sepsis), which is characterized by sepsis with evidence of deleterious

TABLE 8.1. Definitions in sepsis.

Systemic inflammatory response syndrome

Two or more of the following:

Temperature > 38°C or < 36°C

Heart rate > 90 beats/min

Respiratory rate > 20 breaths/min

White blood cell count > 12,000/mm^3, < 4,000/mm^3, or > 10% of immature cells

Sepsis

SIRS plus a documented infection (positive culture)

If culture negative, suspected infection and one of the following:

Significant edema or positive fluid balance (20 ml/kg over 20 h)

Hyperglycemia (plasma glucose > 120 mg/dl) in the absence of diabetes

Inflammatory variables: plasma C-reactive protein > 2 SD above the normal value or plasma procalcitonin > 2SD above the normal value

Mixed venous oxygen saturation (SVO$_2$) > 70%

Cardiac index > 3.5 l/min/M^{23}

Severe sepsis

Sepsis associated with organ dysfunction, hypoperfusion abnormalities, or hypotension

Hypoperfusion abnormalities include, but are not limited to:

Arterial hypoxemia (PaO$_2$/fraction of inspired oxygen (FiO$_2$) ration of < 300 torr)

Acute oliguria (urine output < 0.5 ml/kg/h or 45 mmol/l for at least 2 h)

Creatinine > 2.0 mg/dl

Coagulation abnormalities (international normalized ratio > 1.5 or activated partial thromboplastin time > 60 s)

Thrombocytopenia (platelet count < 100,000)

Hyperbilirubinemia (plasma total bilirubin > 2 mg/dl or 35 mmol/l)

Tissue-perfusion variable: hyperlactatemia (>2 mmol/l)

Hemodynamic variables: arterial hypotension

(systolic blood < 90 mmHg, mean arterial pressure < 70 mmHg, or a systolic blood pressure decrease > 40 mmHg)

Septic shock

Sepsis-induced hypotension despite fluid resuscitation plus hypoperfusion abnormalities consequences of the host response with respect to organ perfusion and/or function, and septic shock, in which sepsis syndrome is associated with hypotension, which persists despite apparently adequate fluid resuscitation.

Pathophysiology of Sepsis

The complex pathological processes underlying sepsis and its progression to septic shock result primarily from host immune dysregulation associated with widespread cellular injury and associated tissue and organ dysfunction – invading microorganisms appear to act as initiators, but may rapidly become bystanders as maladaptive systemic immune responses develop. Why some surgical patients produce prompt protective immunological responses to microbial invasion while others develop overwhelming and refractory septic shock remains unclear.

Regulated innate immune activation involves early recognition of the pathogenic microorganism by an array of immunocompetent cells such as macrophages, dendritic cells, lymphocytes, neutrophils, and endothelial cells. Toll-like receptors are a class of pattern-recognition molecules variably expressed on these cells which are able to bind with whole subsets of pathogens or their breakdown products (pathogen-associated molecular patterns). The Toll-like receptor family is evolutionarily conserved, representing a phylogenetically ancient defense mechanism in multicellular organisms which, unlike acquired immune function, does not rely on previous pathogen exposure in the host. Toll-like receptors mediate cell-signaling mechanisms that control the release of cytokines from cells exposed to pathogens or their products. Cytokines are soluble, low-molecular weight glycoproteins that regulate innate and acquired immune responses to pathogens. They act pleiotropically on multiple target cells, having both paracrine and endocrine effects depending on levels of production. Cytokines are traditionally classified into those that produce pro-inflammatory effects (e.g., TNFα, IL-1, and IL-8) and those that are anti-inflammatory (e.g., IL-10 and TGFβ).

Regulated inflammation, local to the site of pathogen invasion, involves release and amplification of pro-inflammatory mediators that promote activation and tissue recruitment of cells, such as circulating neutrophils that have the capacity to destroy invading pathogens (and surrounding tissue) by release of chemicals such as oxygen radicals. Local activation of other inflammatory systems such as complement, coagulation, and kinin-cascades aids in the effective destruction of pathogens and facilitates an appropriate concentration of the inflammatory processes locally. A careful balanced regulation of pro-and anti-inflammatory cytokines, both temporally and spatially, is thought to limit these processes to the tissue site(s) of invasion, limit tissue injury, and promote healing and resolution. The potential for extensive systemic tissue injury and organ dysfunction is clear if this process becomes severely dysregulated.

The prevailing "canonical" theory of sepsis refers to an uncontrolled systemic inflammatory response to overwhelming infection; death from sepsis is attributable to an overstimulated immune system that produces widespread tissue injury and organ dysfunction. However, most of the evidence for this notion is from rigid animal models of sepsis that do not seem to reflect the veracity of human responses to infection. Indeed, in many animal models of endotoxemia or polymicrobial sepsis, organ dysfunction and/or death is often associated with an early and pronounced pro-inflammatory "cytokine storm," and compounds that block the mediators in these models improve survival. The patterns of systemic cytokine levels in surgical patients with sepsis syndromes suggest that "cytokine storm" is unusual and numerous clinical trials of inflammatory cascade blockade with agents, such as corticosteroids, anti-endotoxin antibodies, TNF antagonism, IL-1 receptor antagonists, and other compounds, have failed to make a significant impact on adult human sepsis syndromes. Observational studies in patients suggest that a dysregulated systemic balance between pro-and anti-inflammatory responses may be more important in terms of the pathogenesis of sepsis rather than the magnitude and character of the initial pro-inflammatory status.

Mapping the inflammatory responses onto the clinical manifestations is troublesome, uncovering our inadequate knowledge of basic mechanisms and the nonspecific diagnostic criteria for clinical recognition of sepsis syndromes. However, the SIRS, or sepsis when infection-related, can be associated with an early systemic pro-inflammatory phenotype usually lasting over a number of days, followed by the development of a counter-regulatory anti-inflammatory syndrome (CARS) characterized by immunosuppression (delayed hypersensitivity, an inability to clear infection, and a predisposition to nosocomial infection). Numerous factors have been implicated in the development of immunosuppression in sepsis including unbalanced anti-inflammatory cytokine production, T-cell anergy and apoptosis-induced loss of adaptive immune system. It is unclear why these events occur and how they are related to initial triggering of immune responses to pathogens. Furthermore, in the critically ill surgical patient, it is also unclear how a complex environment (e.g., surgical tissue injury, anesthesia, blood transfusions, nutritional status, and coexisting medical disease) in association with host genetic factors (e.g. polymorphisms in cytokine genes) may determine the mechanisms of responses to an invading pathogen. However, in the practice of surgical critical care, it is unusual for patients to die from overwhelming SIRS/sepsis resulting from the first infection "hit," but the development of CARS during prolonged critical care is associated with a predisposition to secondary "hits" from nosocomial infection, which is closely associated with the development of "multiorgan dysfunction syndrome" (MODS) and a high chance of death.

Sepsis-Related Organ Dysfunction

During sepsis, the development of organ dysfunction distant from the infection site helps define clinical severity (Table 8.1) and is related to outcome. Dysfunction refers to a phenomenon where organ function is not capable of maintaining homeostasis. When more than one organ system is involved it is characterized as MODS, with outcome being directly related to the number and duration of dysfunctional systems. Sepsis-related MODS is the leading cause of death in non-coronary ICUs. Curiously, survival from septic shock is associated with recovery of organ function to baseline. In addition, postmortem examination of surgical patients dying from septic shock uncovers discordance between histological findings and the degree of organ dysfunction. Alongside emerging evidence for mitochondrial dysfunction associated with sepsis and MODS, this clinical evidence suggests cells may develop a "hibernation" phenomenon in response to progressive sepsis, akin to cell stunning following myocardial ischemia.

While any organ can contribute to sepsis-related MODS, the cardiovascular system is commonly implicated and provides an example of how developing organ dysfunction can drive a vicious cycle of systemic immune activation and tissue injury. Cardiac dysfunction is characterized globally by biventricular myocardial dilatation with persisting tachycardia following fluid resuscitation. Despite a normal to high cardiac output, up to a third of patients with sepsis will have myocardial dysfunction as evidenced at the bedside by decreased responsiveness to fluid resuscitation and catecholamine stimulation. Circulating depressant factors, including TNFα and IL-1β, act in synergy on myocytes through nitric oxide dependent and independent pathways, whereas myocardial hypoperfusion is not associated with this phenomenon. Sepsis is also associated with arteriolar vasodilatation and dysregulation of microcirculatory blood flow, mediated via local nitric oxide production, which can become refractory to therapy. Systemic endothelial activation and barrier dysfunction can result in tissue edema formation. In the absence of early adequate resuscitation in combination with increased insensible fluid losses and with myocardial and vascular dysfunction, maldistribution of perfusion to tissues occurs with the threat of ischemic injury and further organ dysfunction. Widespread fibrin deposition in the microcirculation is associated with the early pro-inflammatory phenotype, producing combined fibrin, platelet, neutrophil, and red blood cell microaggregates, which can promote further tissue ischemia. When fibrin deposition is severe, a state of disseminated intravascular coagulation (DIC) can develop and is associated with increased mortality.

The splanchnic circulation is particularly vulnerable to hypoperfusion in the inadequately resuscitated septic patient. Splanchnic hypoperfusion is associated with gut mucosal ischemia, changes in barrier function, and the potential for translocation of enteric flora into gut mucosal cells and gut-associated lymphoid tissue. There is a potential for the hypoperfused gut to generate a localized inflammatory response to these events and when reperfused can contribute further to systemic inflammatory responses and distant organ injury via drainage from the portal circulation and/or mesenteric lymph channels. Experimental evidence and clinical observation in surgical critical care has not been conclusive in this regard, although there is a consensus that gut ischemia-reperfusion may be an important source of systemic pro-inflammation and is clearly associated with the development of nosocomial second "hit" sepsis during subsequent immunosuppression.

Causes of Sepsis in Surgical Patients

Surgical patients may develop sepsis as a consequence of nosocomial infection, or as a feature of diseases that require surgical treatment. A great deal of acute general surgical practice relates to the management of sepsis due to infection within the peritoneal cavity associated with disease and/or perforation of the gastrointestinal tract, whereas nosocomial sepsis in surgical patients most commonly relates to surgical site infection (SSI), including wounds, pneumonia, urinary tract infections, and blood stream infection, which is frequently (though not necessarily) associated with the use of intravascular devices. The incidence of SSI is regarded as a marker of the quality of surgical care, with national surveillance programs collecting data concerning infection rates, clinical outcome, and causative organisms. The vast majority of sepsis in surgical patients relates to infection with gram-positive (60%) or gram-negative (30%) bacteria, and a small, but an increasingly important proportion of cases relates to infection with opportunist pathogens such as fungi, notably *Candida sp*. The most common gram-positive organisms isolated from surgical patients with sepsis are *Staphylococcus* (*epidermidis* and *aureus*) and *Enterococcus sp.* (notably *Enterococcus faecalis*); Hospital-acquired infection, particularly from strains exhibiting multiple antibiotic resistance, such as MRSA (Methicillin-resistant *Staphylococcus aureus*), or VRE (Vanomycin-resistant *Enterococci*) may be particularly difficult to treat. Common gram-negative organisms isolated from surgical patients with sepsis include *Escherichia coli*, *Klebsiella pneumoniae*, and *Pseudomonas aeruginosa*, while gram-negative sepsis in surgical patients in the ICU may also be due to less invasive opportunist organisms, including *Acinetobacter* and *Enterobacter sp.*

Recognition and Diagnosis of Sepsis

Characteristic features of sepsis include fever (hypothermia occasionally occurs in severe sepsis), tachycardia, and tachypnea, accompanied by leukocytosis (leukopenia is occasionally observed in severe sepsis). Rigors are characteristic of episodic bacteremia, typically seen in intravascular catheter infection, or when infection of a duct system is accompanied by mechanical obstruction, for example, in ascending cholangitis or pyelonephritis. In addition to these nonspecific manifestations of systemic inflammation, there may be features indicative of the site of infection, including signs of peritoneal irritation, urinary tract infection a productive cough, or radiological signs of pulmonary consolidation, or, in the case of soft tissue infection, evidence of cellulitis, erythema, swelling, or even discharge of purulent material from a wound site. In some patients with postoperative abdominal infection, including pelvic and subphrenic abscess, sepsis may develop insidiously, unaccompanied by some or even all of the classical signs of infection. In such cases, patients may present instead with failure to make postoperative progress, jaundice, hypoalbuminemia, hyponatremia, and progressive wasting and catabolism, despite apparently satisfactory nutritional support.

It is important to recognize that aerobic and anaerobic blood cultures, though obligatory in the assessment of the septic patient, are likely to be positive on only approximately 20% of occasions. Overall, less than 50% of patients with severe sepsis have a pathogenic organism identified in blood cultures. Diagnosis in many cases is based, at least initially, on clinical suspicion, with antimicrobial chemotherapy initiated on the basis of an assessment of likely pathogens and modified on the basis of culture of samples taken from the site of infection, and, in the case of surgical infections, from pus especially.

Management of Sepsis — Supportive Medical Therapy

Despite half a century of the establishment and refinement of surgical critical care, mortality from severe sepsis and septic shock has not changed, but the incidence of sepsis is increasing in most countries. However, over the past few years a number of unexpected yet important clinical breakthroughs in adjuvant medical therapy have arisen and have been tested in randomized controlled trials. Many of these advances are currently being adopted by the international critical care community in association with coordinated efforts to assess clinical effectiveness.

Cardiovascular Support

Cardiovascular resuscitation with early goal-directed therapy (EGDT) has been shown to improve survival for emergency department patients presenting with severe sepsis and septic shock. Resuscitation aimed at achieving predetermined values of central venous pressure (CVP) and mean arterial pressure (MAP), urine output and central venous (superior vena cava) oxygen saturation (70%) for the initial 6 h period was able to reduce 28-day mortality, with a number needed to treat (NNT) of six patients. Central venous oxygen saturation was used as a pragmatic surrogate of tissue perfusion and oxygen utilization, with rising values above 70% representing adequate hemodynamic resuscitation. If the threshold value was not achieved with fluid resuscitation to a predetermined CVP, then packed red blood cell transfusions to achieve an hematocrit of at least 30% and/or dobutamine infusion (up to 20 μg/kg/min) were titrated to achieve the central venous oxygen saturation goal.

Modification of the Inflammatory Response

Recombinant activated protein C (rhAPC) infusion (24 μg/kg/h) over 96 h has been shown to be effective in improving 28-day survival in patients at high risk of death (sepsis-induced organ dysfunction) and a low risk of bleeding at inception; NNT of 13 with a minimum of two organ dysfunction. It may be important to define more fully those patients most likely to benefit from rhAPC infusion and patients with single organ dysfunction (however severe), who are within 30 days of surgery, and may be most likely to develop complications of treatment and have substantially reduced clinical benefit. The inflammatory response to sepsis is pro-coagulant in the early stages, with the potential for microcirculatory perfusion abnormalities. rhAPC has endogenous anticoagulant and anti-inflammatory properties, which may explain its efficacy in early severe sepsis and septic shock (Fig. 8.1). Taken together, EGDT in the first 6 h of diagnosis, followed by careful consideration for rhAPC therapy, constitutes an effective global reperfusion strategy for high-risk sepsis and should have a similar priority in critical care as reperfusing the myocardium after acute coronary artery thrombosis. For these approaches to work effectively, emergency medical systems must develop strategies for early recognition of the patient with, or at risk of developing, severe sepsis and septic shock. Unfortunately, the diagnosis of sepsis in critical care is rather nonspecific, particularly as culture-positive sepsis is frequently lacking. The need for specific and sensitive

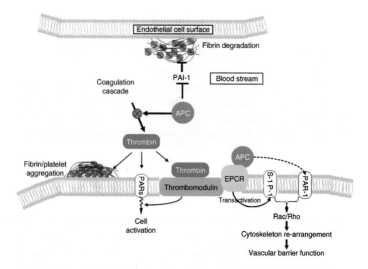

FIGURE 8.1. The Protein C pathway (Reprinted from Macias et al., 2005. With permission).

biomarkers of sepsis, and its severity, has never been more urgent and constitutes a significant scientific challenge.

Administering large-dose intravenous corticosteroids (>300 mg/day of hydrocortisone or equivalent) has been a popular intervention for attempted reversal of refractory hypotension resulting from sepsis, until a more recent meta-analysis reported a worsened prognosis following such interventions; with some notable exceptions in pediatric (meningitis) and adult (severe typhoid and PCP in AIDS) infectious diseases. However, a recent multicenter-randomized controlled trial with patients in severe septic shock showed a significant shock reversal and reduction of 28-day mortality (NNT = 10) when patients with relative adrenal insufficiency (defined as post-ACTH cortisol rise ≥9 μg/dl) received lower-dose "replacement" steroids. Routine low-dose steroids cannot be recommended at this time for sepsis until a number of important questions that were raised by this study are addressed: how is adrenal insufficiency diagnosed in sepsis, what constitutes "low-dose" steroids, and what are the results of a study in patients with sepsis in extremis generalizable to a broader population of critically ill septic patients? These questions are being addressed currently by the international community and further guidance is awaited.

Metabolic and Nutritional Support

A large single-center trial of "tight glycemia" control in postoperative surgical critical care patients (predominantly cardiac surgery) showed improved 28-day survival (NNT = 11) and significant reductions in sepsis-related complications. In the intervention, blood glucose was maintained in the range 80–110 mg/dl (4.4–6.1 mmol/l) using a titrated continuous intravenous insulin infusion. The control of blood sugar appeared to be more important than the amount of infused insulin, but this remains to be formally tested. In addition, other metabolic effects such as a change in circulating lipid profiles may be significant. There is a potential for hypoglycemia, although careful and repeated glucose monitoring in a well-staffed critical care unit, alongside a nutrition protocol that promotes early continuous feeding, can limit these events and ameliorate any potential adverse risk to the patient. Studies aimed at determining the efficacy of less intensive glycemia control may help further reduce any risk of insulin infusions. Another large study at the same center has recently extended the "tight glycemia" approach to medical intensive care and did not replicate the survival advantage in the intervention group on an intention-to-treat basis. At present, the concept and scientific basis for "tight glycemia" control is in evolution and should probably be reserved for critically ill surgical patients in the ICU.

Sepsis is a catabolic state, associated with profound resistance to the anabolic effects of insulin and muscle wasting, despite aggressive nutritional support. Attempts to modify the hormonal environment to promote anabolism using recombinant human growth hormone (rhGH), while attractive in theory, were abandoned when it became clear that this approach resulted in increased mortality, possibly because of

GH-induced insulin resistance and the resulting hyperglycemia and increased risk of sepsis. While there has been considerable debate concerning the optimal route for nutritional
support in patients with sepsis and the controversial role of
immune-enhancing feeds, pragmatic trials have shown that
the route of feeding is probably less important than ensuring
adequate (but not excessive) provision of calories and nitrogen in a safe manner, tailored to the patient's individual
requirements and the ability of their gastrointestinal tract to
cope with enteral feeding. Nutritional support should not be
expected to reverse catabolism in the presence of ongoing
sepsis and dealing with the source of sepsis is one of the most
valuable interventions from the nutritional perspective.

Antimicrobial Chemotherapy

Appropriate antibiotic use in sepsis provides a major challenge to the surgeon, critical care physician, and microbiolo-
gist because scientific evidence for any particular approach is
lacking. In many cases, early use of broad-spectrum antibiotics guided by surveillance-driven local policy against the suspected pathogen(s) in a given clinical sepsis scenario would
be considered best practice. Continued laboratory and
clinical surveillance should then allow de-escalation and
fine-tuning of antimicrobial therapies in order to maximize
efficacy and limit drug-induced organ injury and superinfec-
tion with multiresistant pathogens. However, in recent years,
evidence for adjuvant selective gut decontamination of critically ill patients in intensive care has been growing. There are
now two meta-analyses which confirm survival advantage by
providing a combination of topical and parenteral broad-
spectrum antibiotics aimed at early gut microflora eradica-
tion, thereby limiting the role of the gut as a pro-inflammatory
organ and source of second "hit" infection during critical
care. Despite the compelling evidence for efficacy, early
selective gut decontamination in critical illness has not
been universally adopted, primarily because of concerns
for the development of antimicrobial resistance — evidence

for which has not arisen in the meta-analyses. It remains to be seen if the international community reconsiders its approach to the gut microflora which is carried into ICUs by the host.

Management of Sepsis — Principles of Surgical Therapy

In many surgical patients, prompt surgical intervention is of paramount importance in treating sepsis. Although aggressive resuscitation and antimicrobial chemotherapy are essential, a successful outcome of treatment is unlikely unless source control is achieved. Devitalized or necrotic tissue should be removed, the pus drained and sent for culture, and the results used to modify further antibiotic therapy, if appropriate (see above). In many cases of abdominal infection, this can be achieved by percutaneous drainage, under ultrasound guidance without exposing the patient to the additional risk of multiple organ failure syndrome (MOFS) associated with the second "hit" of further surgery. Where source control, however, requires resection or removal of the focus of infection (e.g., a perforated viscus or a leaking anastomosis), this is better accomplished by surgical means. Studies of patients with intra-abdominal sepsis have shown, for example, that ability to eradicate the abdominal septic focus is the single most important determinant of survival, and failure to do so on the first occasion is associated with a significantly increased mortality, which increases stepwise with each successive trip to the theater, and that the prognosis is especially poor if septic shock develops prior to treatment.

The general principles of surgical intervention are to establish adequate drainage of infection and to excise necrotic or devitalized tissue. Obstruction to the biliary or urinary tract must be relieved by radiological, endoscopic, or surgical means. Leakage from the gastrointestinal tract should be dealt with by exteriorization wherever possible. In patients with severe abdominal sepsis, up to 30% of patients exhibit continuing evidence of infection after aggressive surgical intervention, typified by intra-abdominal abscess formation, often with multiple small abscesses between loops of small intestine (tertiary peritonitis). The role of planned relaparotomy, as opposed to laparotomy on demand (in relation to deterioration in oxygenation, organ function, and inotrope requirements), in such cases remains controversial, but case–control studies have shown that planned relaparotomy does not appear to reduce mortality significantly and may increase secondary complications, including the incidence of intestinal fistula. In severe cases of tertiary peritonitis, where sepsis frequently coexists with abdominal hypertension, management may necessitate leaving the abdomen open (laparostomy) to facilitate drainage of the septic focus and planned, staged reconstructive surgery of the gastrointestinal tract and abdominal wall after recovery.

Selected Readings

Bone RC, Balk RA, Cerra FB (1992) Definitions for sepsis and organ failure and guidelines for the use of innovative therapies in sepsis. The ACCP/SCCM consensus conference committee. Chest 101:1644–55

Carlson GL, Irving MH (1997) Infection: recognition and management of infection in surgical patients. In: Hanson G (ed.) Critical care of the surgical patient — a companion to Bailey and Loves' surgery. Chapman & Hall, London, pp. 273–290

Dellinger RP, Carlet JM, Masur H, et al. (2004) Surviving Sepsis Campaign guidelines for management of severe sepsis and septic shock. Crit Care Med 32(3):858–873

Hotchkiss RS, Karl IE (2003) The pathophysiology and treatment of sepsis. N Engl J Med 348(2):138–150

Levy MM, Fink MP, Marshall JC, et al. (2003) 2001 SCCM/ ESICM/ ACCP/ATS/SIS International Sepsis Definitions Conference. Crit Care Med 31(4):1250–1256

Macias WL, Yan SB, Williams MD, et al. (2005) New insights into the protein C pathway: potential implications for the biological activities of Drotrecogin alfa (activated). Crit Care 9 (Suppl 4):S38–S45

National nosocomial infection surveillance (1998) Systems report, data. Summary from October 1986–April 1998, issued June 1998. Am J Infect Control 26:522–533

Rivers E, Nguyen B, Havstad S, et al. (2001) Early goal-directed therapy in the treatment of severe sepsis and septic shock. N Engl J Med 345(19):1368–1377

Singer M, De Santis V, Vitale D, Jeffcoate W (2004) Multi-organ failure is an adaptive, endocrine-mediated, metabolic response to over-whelming systemic inflammation. Lancet 364(9433):545–548

van den Berghe G, Wouters P, Weekers F, et al. (2001) Intensive insulin therapy in critically ill patients. N Engl J Med 345(19):1359–1367

9
Neurologic Physiology: The Brain and Its Response to Injury

Mamerhi O. Okor and James M. Markert

Pearls and Pitfalls

- Early clinical recognition and radiographic diagnosis are key initial steps in the management of head injury.
- Once a surgical lesion has been ruled out in a severely head-injured patient, aggressive medical management should be instituted. Medical management primarily constitutes supportive therapy aimed at preventing secondary insults to the brain, which should include the detection and treatment of raised intracranial pressure (ICP).
- In the event that first-line therapy for the management of elevated ICPs is unsuccessful, "second-tier" therapy may be cautiously applied.
- Lack of an aggressive initial approach to the head-injured patient can lead to an exacerbation of the initial injury due to potentially avoidable secondary injury – an inadequate resuscitation can lead to superimposed hypoxic or ischemic injury, and delayed institution of measures to combat increased ICP can result in increases in local tissue pressures and local ischemia, or even avoidable herniation syndromes.
- A poor neurologic exam in the setting of an initially normal-appearing computed tomography (CT) scan may be due to toxic/metabolic issues, but also can be a result of a hypoxic injury or diffuse axonal injury (DAI).

K.I. Bland et al. (eds.), *Critical Care Surgery*,
DOI 10.1007/978-1-84996-378-7_9,
© Springer-Verlag London Limited 2011

- An early accurate neurologic assessment can prevent the clinician from delaying the diagnosis of an intracranial mass lesion that may require immediate operative intervention, particularly if a unilateral fixed and dilated pupil is present, or a patient has a marked hemiparesis.
- Patients in whom such an exam is not possible due to pharmacologic paralysis before such an assessment can be undertaken, require an urgent head CT to avoid missing such a diagnosis.
- Overuse of hyperventilation (prolonged periods of $PaCO_2$ of 25 mmHg or less) can result in rebound intracranial hypertension; $PaCO_2$ should generally be kept in the 30–35 mmHg range. Serum osmolarity should be maintained below 310–320 to minimize the risk of renal injury in the setting of prolonged mannitol administration, and switching to hyperosmolar saline use in these patients can decrease this risk.
- Avoidable use of pharmacologic paralysis can lead to sepsis, pneumonia, and increased ICU stays.

Classification of Brain Injury

Closed head injury can be classified based on severity (mild, moderate, or severe) which is determined largely by Glasgow Coma Scale scoring; mechanism (missile or blunt); and pathology (primary or secondary). A prompt and thorough initial neurologic assessment is crucial in determining the nature of a patient's injury and instituting the appropriate treatment protocol.

Missile Injuries

Missile injuries can be classified as depressed, penetrating, or perforating. In *depressed injuries*, the missile fails to penetrate the skull but produces a depressed skull fracture and/or causes a contusional injury to the underlying brain. Brain damage is therefore focal, and consciousness is rarely altered for long. In *penetrating injuries*, the missile enters the cranial cavity but does not leave it. If the object is small and sharp, and penetration is limited, little direct injury to the skull and brain may occur. The damage is focal, and the patient seldom loses consciousness. However, the missile may penetrate deeply enough to damage vital structures. Penetration through multiple lobes, both hemispheres, the ventricular system, or posterior fossa involvement by the missile will all produce more extensive damage. Even simple penetrating head injuries may allow infection, meningitis, or cerebral abscesses to develop. In a penetrating injury, the missile (usually a bullet) passes and exits the brain but does not leave the skull, resulting in a penetrating brain wound. If the bullet exits the head, the injury is called a *perforating head injury*. The exit wound in the skull is characteristically larger than the entry wound. Low-velocity missiles rarely exit the skull, although they often produce multiple destructive tracts through the brain in which there may be bone fragments, soft tissues, and clothing. Although a high-velocity bullet may pass through the head without causing impairment of consciousness, brain damage in these circumstances tend to be severe and extensive, likely due to the shockwaves generated by the missile. Any missile injury can result in the formation of a hematoma, which can further complicate injury management and patient outcome.

Blunt Injuries

Blunt injuries frequently result in scalp lacerations, skull fractures, contusions, subdural hematomas (SDHs), epidural hematomas (EDHs), and axonal shear injuries. *Scalp lacerations* can be of considerable importance as sources of blood loss and indications of the site of injury. If there is an associated depressed skull fracture, scalp lacerations represent a potential avenue for intracranial infection.

Skull fractures may involve the cranial vault or skull base and may be classified as linear or depressed. The frequency of skull fractures appears to correlate with the severity of head injury. Patients with a fracture have a much higher incidence of intracranial hematoma than patients without a fracture. A depressed skull fracture is considered to be compound if an associated scalp laceration extending through the pericranium is present, and penetrating if a dural laceration exists. Depressed fractures are more likely to provide potential routes for intracranial infections than linear fractures, and are associated with an increased incidence of post-traumatic epilepsy. Skull base fractures may also be complicated by intracranial infections, as organisms may spread from the air sinuses or the middle ear, especially in the setting of an undiagnosed or untreated cerebrospinal fluid (CSF) fistula (CSF rhinorrhea or otorrhea).

Intracranial hemorrhage is a common complication of head injury and is the most common cause of clinical deterioration and death in patients who experienced a lucid interval after injury. Intracranial injury may be subdivided into extra-axial hematomas, which include EDHs, SDHs, subarachnoid hemorrhages, and intracerebral hematomas which arise within the parenchyma of the brain. Although intracranial hematomas can be identified on initial CT evaluation, the severity of its clinical manifestations along with the potential for delayed neurologic deterioration are due in large part to the time it takes for the hematoma to attain a size sufficient to cause brain distortion and herniation, as well as the development of associated edema. Expanding hematomas should be distinguished from delayed hematomas, which are described as lesions that occur more than 24 h after the time of injury that are not evident on initial imaging studies.

Most intracranial hematomas develop within the first 48 h after injury, but SDHs may also be subacute (2–14 days after injury) or chronic (more than 14 days after injury).

Epidural hematomas or EDHs (Fig. 9.1) often result from hemorrhage from a meningeal artery, most often a branch of the middle meningeal artery, and are associated with overlying skull fractures in 90% of adult patients. The incidence of skull fractures is lower in children with EDHs. EDHs occur most often in the temporal region but 25% occur elsewhere, such as in the

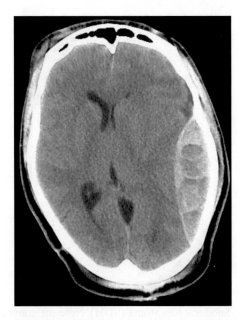

FIGURE 9.1. Epidural hematoma. Note the lentiform nature and the significant mass effect on the ventricular system, with left to right shift. Most of these lesions arise from damage to the middle meningeal artery or other dural vessels, and are often associated with skull fractures.

frontal and parietal regions or within the posterior fossa, where they may occur as a result of venous sinus injury. Occasionally, these hematomas are multiple. As the hematoma enlarges, it strips the dural from the skull, forming an elliptical mass that is limited by the dural investment into the calvarial sutures. In patients who experience a lucid interval, there is often little evidence of other types of brain injury. If however, the patient has been in a coma from the time of the original injury, other types of brain injury are likely to be present. Isolated EDHs of <30 ml in volume infrequently cause an alteration in the level of consciousness or a focal neurologic deficit.

Subdural hematomas or SDHs (Fig. 9.2) are brought on by the rupture of the bridging veins that connect cortical veins

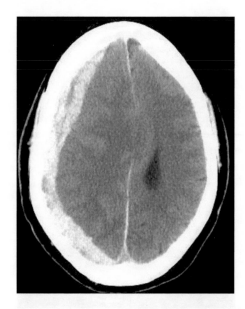

FIGURE 9.2. Subdural hematoma (SDH). Note the convex shape of the lesion. SDHs are usually associated with acute underlying brain injury and generally have a worse prognosis than epidural hematomas (EDHs).

to dural venous sinuses or from a laceration in a cortical artery. Subdural veins are sensitive to the rate at which they are deformed by acceleration (strain-sensitive). The general morbidity and mortality rates are greater for subdural hematomas than for EDHs because of the higher incidence of concurrent brain damage. SDHs are classified by their appearance, classically on CT imaging, as follows: acute when the hematoma is composed of clotted blood that appears hyperdense to brain tissue on noncontrast head CT; subacute when composed of a mixture of clotted and fluid blood that appears isodense to brain tissue; or chronic when composed purely of liquefied blood and proteins mixed with CSF that appears hypodense to brain tissue. The clotted blood remains for at least 48 h and sometimes several days. The transition to a more fluid blood is largely due to the action of fibrinolytic enzymes that dissolve the clot. These enzymes start this dissolution within 72–96 h after clot formation. After about 3 weeks, no clot remains. In about 25% of patients who undergo evacuation of an acute SDH, acute brain edema occurs in the hemisphere underlying the clot and portends a poor prognosis.

Cerebral contusions have long since been considered the hallmark of head injury. Contusions occur characteristically in the frontal and temporal poles and on the inferior surfaces of the frontal and temporal lobes where the brain tissue comes in contact with the protuberances at the skull base. In early stages, they are hemorrhagic and swollen, but with time they evolve into shrunken gliotic scars. Because the damage is focal, patients with severe contusions may have an uneventful recovery from head injury, provided that they do not develop complications leading to other types of brain damage and that they do not sustain diffuse axonal injury (DAI) at the time of original injury. Contusions can be further subdivided into fracture contusions, coup contusions, contra-coup contusions, and herniation contusions. Fracture contusions occur at the site of a fracture and are particularly severe in the frontal lobe. Coup contusions occur at the site of injury in the absence of a fracture. Contra-coup contusions in the brain occur diametrically opposed to the point of injury as a result of brain movement within the calvarium. Herniation contusions occur when the medial parts of the temporal lobes are impacted against the edge of the tentorium, or the cerebellar tonsils are impacted against the foramen magnum at the site of the injury.

Intracerebral hematomas (Fig. 9.3) are found in approximately 15% of all patients who sustain fatal head injuries. These hematomas may be single or multiple, and occur primarily in the frontal and temporal regions. They most likely result from a direct rupture of intrinsic cerebral blood vessel in relation to contusions at the time of injury.

Diffuse axonal injury, or DAI, occurs when the head and brain are subject to severe rotational forces, and is characterized by the shearing of nerve fibers at the moment of injury.

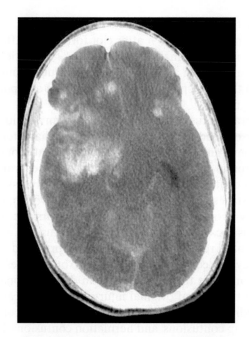

FIGURE 9.3. Multiple intraparenchymal hematomas. These lesions arise within the parenchyma of the brain itself and indicate a significant injury to the brain itself. They can produce mass effect and also may evolve over the days post-injury to produce edema, which may produce increases in ICP if the hematoma is not evacuated surgically.

The clinical presentation of DAI remains varied. Patients may present with brief periods of altered consciousness or may remain in a coma for extended periods of time. In severe cases, patients with DAI are left in a persistent vegetative state or may expire depending on the severity of concurrent secondary injury. Patients with DAI have a statistically lower incidence of lucid intervals, skull fractures, cerebral contusions, intracerebral hematomas, and evidence of elevated intracranial pressures (ICPs). In the absence of magnetic resonance imaging (MRI) or characteristic CT findings, the diagnosis of DAI is largely exclusionary, encompassing a spectrum of patients with severe closed head injury and a paucity of findings on noncontrast head CT. In its most severe form, DAI is characterized by focal lesions in the corpus callosum, focal lesions in the dorsolateral aspect of the rostral brainstem, and evidence of diffuse injury to axons. These focal lesions may be evident as petechial hemorrhages on a noncontrast CT scan. Since the advent of the MRI with its high sensitivity for parenchymal injury, the definition of DAI has been expanded to include patients with nonhemorrhagic areas of T2 signal within the white matter or at the gray–white junction.

Secondary Brain Injury

An increase in the volume of all or part of the brain is common in patients who sustain severe blunt head injury. The resultant edema may be severe enough to raise the ICP and cause death from brain shift, herniation, and secondary damage to the brainstem. The brain swelling is largely due to an increase in cerebral blood volume (congestive brain swelling) or water content of the brain tissue (cerebral edema). Brain swelling can be classified into three types: swelling adjacent to contusions, diffuse swelling of one cerebral hemisphere, and diffuse swelling of both cerebral hemispheres.

Swelling of the brain adjacent to contusions is common and is due to physical disruption of the tissue with damage to the blood brain barrier and loss of normal physiologic autoregulation of arterioles. Water and electrolytes leak into the brain tissue and spread into the adjacent white matter.

Diffuse swelling of one cerebral hemisphere is most often seen in association with an ipsilateral acute SDH. When the hematoma is evacuated, the brain simply expands to fill the space created. This is attributed to engorgement of a nonreactive vascular bed with regional loss of normal autoregulation and can be accompanied by superimposed ischemia. The initiation of swelling results from cerebral vasodilatation followed by a breakdown of the blood brain barrier, leading to cerebral edema. Some authorities have suggested that in a patient in whom a SDH is not clinically apparent until 2–3 days after the injury, the progressive development of brain swelling is more likely the cause of clinical deterioration and elevated ICP than hematoma expansion.

Diffuse swelling of both cerebral hemispheres tends to occur in young patients. The pathogenesis of this type of brain damage is unclear, but in the pediatric population, dysfunctional autoregulation leading to a loss of vasomotor tone and consequent vasodilatation may contribute to the swelling. If the vasodilatation persists, the blood brain barrier may become defective and true edema may result.

Superimposed ischemic and hypoxic brain damage is common in patients that sustain severe blunt traumatic head injury. It is significantly more common in patients who sustain a clinical episode of hypotension or hypoxia (systolic blood pressure (SBP) < 80 mmHg for at least 15 min, or a PaO_2 < 50 mmHg at some time after injury) than in those who do not. Such damage is also more common in patients who experience high ICPs. A significant correlation also exists between ischemic brain damage in patients who sustain blunt head injury and arterial spasm. The presence of ischemic damage in arterial watershed areas suggests that the patient may sustain a period of cerebral perfusion failure due to an episode of hypotension. Ischemic damage is thus another potential cause of traumatic coma in the absence of an intracranial mass lesion. Such damage is also a frequent finding in patients who remain vegetative or severely disabled after sustaining a head injury.

Evaluation and Management of Severe Closed Head Injury

Early clinical recognition and radiographic diagnosis are key initial steps in the management of head injury. Also important is the need for serial clinical and radiographic assessment of the head-injured patient as the primary thrust of management should be geared towards determining whether the patient has a lesion that requires urgent neurosurgical attention. The initial neurologic assessment of a head-injured patient should be prompt and aimed at evaluating the patient's level of consciousness, as well as symmetry of neurologic function from head to toe. This should include a determination of the patient's Glasgow Coma Scale (GCS) score, a cranial nerve exam that evaluates pupillary function, extraocular movements, facial symmetry, and vital cranial nerve reflexes, as well as a good motor exam. A thorough motor examination, however, may be difficult owing to the presence of other systemic injury, other ongoing diagnostic and therapeutic maneuvers, and lack of patient cooperation. The data acquired are an important indicator of the significance and severity of possible cerebral and brainstem compression. In a pharmacologically paralyzed patient, the pupillary exam encompasses the entirety of the neurologic examination and must be performed in an accurate and serial fashion.

A prompt radiographic evaluation with a noncontrast head CT scan should follow the neurologic assessment, but may be delayed depending on the patient's resuscitative needs and the resources of the treating facility. The identification of a mass lesion or significant alteration in GCS should prompt an urgent neurosurgical consultation.

Surgical Management

In 2006, the Congress of Neurologic Surgeons formed guidelines for the surgical management of traumatic brain injury (TBI). The guidelines are briefly summarized as follows:

- EDHs > 30 ml in volume should be surgically evacuated regardless of the patient's GCS score. Patients with an acute EDH in coma (GCS < 9) with pupillary asymmetry should undergo surgical evacuation as soon as possible.
- An acute SDH with thickness > 10 mm or a midline shift > 5 mm on CT scan should be surgically evacuated regardless of GCS score. All patients with acute SDH in coma

should undergo ICP monitoring. A comatose patient with an SDH < 10 mm thickness and a midline shift < 5mm should undergo surgical evacuation if the GCS score decreases between the time of injury and hospital admission by two or more points, and/or the patient presents with asymmetric or fixed and dilated pupils, and/or the ICP exceeds 20 mmHg.

- Patients with parenchymal mass lesions (contusions and intracerebral hematomas) and signs of progressive neurological deterioration referable to the lesion, medically refractory intracranial hypertension, or signs of mass effect on CT scan should be treated operatively. Patients' GCS scores of 6–8 with frontal or temporal lesions < 20 ml in volume with a midline shift of at least 5 mm and/or cisternal compression on CT scan, and patients with any lesion > 50 cc in volume should be treated operatively.

Medical Management

In the absence of a surgical lesion, rapid and aggressive medical management should be instituted. The medical management of the head-injured patient is directed largely at supportive therapy, as well as the prevention and treatment of the secondary effects of traumatic head injury which manifest primarily as raised ICP.

We tend to err on the side of initiating aggressive treatment of patients with presumed severe TBI (GCS < 8) before a radiographic diagnosis is made because we believe that the rapid initiation of therapeutic measures is paramount in preventing insults that may result from the secondary effects of traumatic head injury. Our treatment strategy is based largely on guidelines set forth by the Brain Trauma Foundation and Joint Section on Neurotrauma and Critical Care of the AANS in 2000 entitled Management and Prognosis of Severe Traumatic Brain Injury, and is summarized below. While much of this summary comes directly from these guidelines, we have indicated our favored management approaches wherever appropriate.

General Care and Supportive Measures

Hypotension (SBP < 90 mmHg) and hypoxia (apnea, cyanosis, and oxygen (O_2) saturation < 90% in the field or a PaO_2 < 60 mmHg) must be monitored, and avoided if possible or corrected immediately in severe TBI patients. The mean arterial pressure (MAP) should be maintained above 90 mmHg through the infusion of fluids, and judicious use of vasopressors if necessary. Patients who are unable to maintain their airway or remain hypoxemic despite supplemental O_2, must have their airway secured, preferably by endotracheal intubation. Central venous pressure and invasive blood pressure monitoring are mandatory. A Swan-Ganz catheter should be considered strongly in patients with cardiopulmonary disease or those requiring extensive vasopressor therapy. Red blood cell rheology, as well as the oxygen-carrying capacity of blood, should be optimized by maintaining a hematocrit between 30% and 34%. All efforts should be made to avoid hyperglycemia as this can be common in head-injured patients, and may aggravate cerebral edema and secondary injury. Strict glycemic control with frequent blood glucose checks and treatment of elevated levels (<150 mg/dl) with subcutaneous or IV insulin is strongly encouraged. As a treatment option, anticonvulsants may be used to prevent early post-traumatic seizures (seizures occurring within 7 days of the initial injury) in patients at high risk for seizures following head injury. Prophylactic therapy should last no longer than 7 days. Phenytoin and carbamazepine have been shown to be effective in preventing early post-traumatic seizures. However, there is not sufficient evidence to demonstrate that the prevention of early post-traumatic seizures improves outcome following head injury. The use of steroids is not recommended for improving outcome or reducing ICP in patients with severe TBI, as it has not been shown to improve outcome and results in increased complication rates.

Intracranial Pressure Monitoring

ICP monitoring is appropriate in patients with GCS scores of 3–8 after adequate cardiopulmonary resuscitation and abnormal head CT that reveals hematomas, edema, contusions, or compressed basal cisterns. It is appropriate in patients with GCS scores of 3–8 with normal head CT if two or more of the following are noted on admission: age > 40 years, unilateral or bilateral posturing, SBP < 90 mmHg. It is not routinely indicated in patients with mild (GCS 13–15) to moderate (GCS 9–12) head injury; however, a physician may choose to monitor ICP in certain conscious patients with traumatic mass lesions. In the current state of technology, the ventricular catheter connected to an external strain gauge is the most accurate, low-cost, and reliable method of monitoring ICP. It also allows therapeutic CSF drainage. Parenchymal ICP monitoring is similar to ventricular ICP monitoring, but has the potential for measurement drift. Subarachnoid, subdural, and epidural monitors are currently less accurate. The authors' monitor of choice is the ventricular catheter for reasons expressed above. However, in patients with small ventricles, we elect to place a parenchymal monitor if attempts at ventricular cannulation are unsuccessful.

Management of Elevated Intracranial Pressure

Elevations in ICP are tolerated poorly in head injury patients compared with normal individuals because of concomitant dysfunctional autoregulation, brain swelling, and underlying hypoxic ischemic damage (Table 9.1). The intracranial cavity consists of CSF, blood, and brain parenchyma. Following head injury, several mechanisms are set in motion in an attempt to counteract ICP elevations in accordance with the Monroe-Kellie doctrine. Initially, CSF volume is reduced by

TABLE 9.1. Outline of management strategy to treat elevated ICP.

First-line therapy	*Positional changes*
	Maintain head of bed at 30–45°
	Keep neck straight
	Avoid constrictive devices about cervical spine
	Control PaCO$_2$
	Mild hyperventilation
	(maintain PaCO$_2$ between 30–35 mmHg)
	Hyperosmolar therapy
	Mannitol
	Hypertonic saline
	Sedation
	Diprivan (Propofol)
	Lorazepam (Ativan)
	Midazolam (Versed)
	Chemical paralysis
Second-line therapy	*Aggressive hyperventilation*
	(maintain PaCO$_2$ < 30 mmHg; short duration only)
	High-dose barbiturate therapy
	Decompressive craniectomy

displacement of CSF from the intracranial to the spinal compartment, as well as increased CSF resorption. Continued increases in ICP are compensated for by decreases in the intracranial volume by venous compression. If the ICP continues to rise, however, compensatory mechanisms are exhausted, intracranial compliance decreases, and, as a result, smaller changes in volume lead to larger elevations of ICP. ICP treatment should be initiated at an upper threshold of

20 mmHg. Interpretation and treatment of ICP based on any threshold should be corroborated by frequent clinical examination and cerebral perfusion pressure (CPP) data, which is determined by calculating the difference between the MAP and the ICP. CPP should be maintained at a minimum of 60 mmHg. It remains a crude but rapid estimation of blood flow to the brain. If available, more sophisticated determinants of cerebral blood flow (CBF) may be employed. It is important to note that ICP elevations above 20 mmHg are more deleterious to head trauma patients than decreases in CPP below 60 mmHg, and higher CPPs are not as protective in patients with elevated ICPs. Thus every effort should be made to keep the ICP below 20 mmHg.

Elevations in ICP are initially treated with elevation of the patient's head to 30°, mild hyperventilation maintaining the PaCO2 between 30 and 35 mmHg, CSF drainage, hyperosmolar therapy with mannitol or 3% sodium chloride, sedation with Diprivan (Propofol), lorazepam (Ativan), midazolam (Versed) and/or morphine, and chemical paralysis. The elevation of the patient's head of bed up to 30–45° while keeping the neck straight and avoiding any constricting devices around the cervical region, helps facilitate venous drainage without compromising the arterial blood supply. Mild hyperventilation results in a decrease in $PaCO_2$, which ultimately leads to cerebral vasoconstriction and a decrease in CBF followed by a decrease in ICP. Mild hyperventilation therapy ($PaCO_2$ between 30 and 35 mmHg) may be useful during long periods of refractory intracranial hypertension. In the presence of increased ICPs, prolonged aggressive hyperventilation therapy ($PaCO_2$ < 25 mmHg) should be avoided in severe TBI given its effects on cerebral perfusion and potential for cerebral ischemia, especially in the first 24 h following injury when cerebral blood flows. For the same reason, prophylactic hyperventilation therapy should be avoided if possible. However, more aggressive hyperventilation therapy ($PaCO_2$ < 30 mmHg) may be necessary for brief periods when there is acute neurologic deterioration.

Mannitol is effective for control of raised ICP after severe TBI. Effective doses range from 0.25 to 1 g/kg body weight.

The indications for use of mannitol prior to ICP monitoring are signs of transtentorial herniation or progressive neurologic deterioration not attributable to extracranial complaints. The patient's fluid status must be monitored closely, especially when there is concomitant use of diuretics to ensure the avoidance of hypovolemia and hypotension. Mannitol increases the osmolality of blood acutely, which helps withdraw water from the brain into the bloodstream. It is effective only with an intact blood brain barrier, however, and a delayed rebound phenomenon of elevated ICP can occur secondary to the entry of mannitol into the brain. It also functions as a free radical scavenger and decreases blood viscosity, which transiently increases CBF and triggers cerebral vasoconstriction, which in turn acutely lowers ICP. Serum osmolarity should be kept below 320 mOsm due to concerns for renal failure. Intermittent boluses may be more effective than a continuous infusion of mannitol. Hypertonic saline (3% or 7.5% NaCl; some investigators use even higher concentrations) is an accepted alternative to mannitol. Like mannitol, it is effective in treating elevated ICP, and has favorable effects of cerebral perfusion and red blood cell rheology. However, it has a more favorable side-effect profile and is the authors' preferred choice for hyperosmolar therapy in the setting of prolonged (>3–5 days) intracranial hypertension.

Precipitous spikes in ICP should be evaluated with a noncontrast head CT scan. This is aimed at detecting a surgical lesion before it contributes to refractory intracranial hypertension.

"Second-Line" Therapy for Persistent Elevated Intracranial Pressure

In the event that the above-described measures are unsuccessful in addressing elevated ICPs, "second-line" therapy may be instituted. These measures are so named because they are either effective therapies with significant risks or are unproven in terms of benefit on outcome. They include aggressive hyperventilation, high-dose barbiturate therapy, hypothermia, and decompressive craniectomy.

High-dose barbiturate therapy may be considered in hemodynamically salvageable, severe TBI patients with intracranial hypertension refractory to maximum medical and surgical ICP-lowering therapy. The benefits of barbiturates stem from vasoconstriction in normal areas (shunting blood to ischemic brain tissue), decreased metabolic demand for oxygen (CMRO2) with accompanying reduction of CBF, free radical scavenging, reduced intracellular calcium, and lysosomal stabilization. The primary side effect is hypotension due to barbiturate-induced direct myocardial depression and reduction of sympathetic tone, which leads to peripheral vasodilatation.

Induced hypothermia carries many systemic side effects including pneumonia, thrombocytopenia, pancreatitis, renal failure, and myocardial depression. Whole-body temperature reductions are slowly giving way to focal cerebral hypothermia, which appears to have a lower side-effect profile.

Decompressive craniectomy involves the removal of a portion of the calvaria with or without the resection of large areas of contused brain. This measure remains controversial, as results of clinical studies to date have been inconsistent and remain under investigation.

Selected Readings

Bullock MR, et al. (2000) Guidelines for the management of severe traumatic brain injury. American Association of Neurologic Surgeons, Joint Section on Neurotrauma and Critical Care & Traumatic Brain Trauma Foundation, New York

Bullock MR, et al. (2006) Guidelines for the surgical management of traumatic brain injury. Neurosurgery 58(Suppl 3):S2–vi

Lyons MK, Meyer FB (1990) Cerebrospinal fluid physiology and the management of increased intracranial pressure. Mayo Clinic Proc 65:684–707

Rea GL, Rockwold GL (1983) Barbiturate therapy in uncontrolled intracranial hypertension. Neurosurgery; 12:401–404

Tindall GT, Cooper PR, Barrow DL (1996) The practice of neurosurgery, Vol 2. William & Wilkins, Baltimore, MD, pp 1385–1425

Wilkins RH, Rengachary SS (eds) (1996) Neurosurgery, 2nd edn 3 vols. McGraw-Hill, New York, pp 2624–2634

10
Pulmonary Embolism

Lisa K. McIntyre and Lorrie A. Langdale

Pearls and Pitfalls

- Clinical presentation is variable.
- Hypoxemia, respiratory alkalosis, and tachypnea are common but not diagnostic.
- Assessment of clinical risk is crucial to determine the degree of diagnostic testing.
- Spiral CT angiogram of the chest is a cost-effective and accurate initial diagnostic study.
- Ventilation-perfusion scanning is an acceptable study for patients with a contraindication to CT.
- The finding of a DVT with duplex scanning can confirm the diagnosis of PE when the clinical presentation and other diagnostic tests are indeterminate; a negative duplex, however, is insufficient to rule out the diagnosis of PE.
- Initial treatment depends on the degree of physiologic compromise:

  - In hemodynamically stable patients, anticoagulation with unfractionated or low molecular weight heparin is the treatment of choice.
  - In hemodynamically unstable patients, thrombolysis or embolectomy should be considered.

K.I. Bland et al. (eds.), *Critical Care Surgery*,
DOI 10.1007/978-1-84996-378-7_10,
© Springer-Verlag London Limited 2011

- Vena cava filters are indicated for patients with contraindications for anticoagulation or failure of anticoagulation.
- Prevention and prophylaxis strategies are dependent on individual risk factors.

Introduction

Despite heightened awareness and advances in technology, the nonspecific clinical presentation of pulmonary embolism continues to pose a diagnostic and management challenge. In autopsy studies by Legere and co-authors, pulmonary emboli (PE) were detected in more than 25% of deaths; 70% of these cases were not clinically apparent prior to the patient's demise. Overall, PE complicates the course of approximately 10% of patients with deep venous system thrombosis (DVT). Thrombi involving the lower extremities proximal to the popliteal fossa present the highest risk. More distal clots are associated with emboli in up to 13% of patients, but as many as 50% of those with documented PE have no leg symptoms or identifiable source of clot. In addition, approximately 10% of upper extremity thrombi embolize to the pulmonary vasculature, an incidence that is further increased when thrombi are associated with central venous catheters. Although the majority of emboli do not result in death, fatalities most often occur within hours of the initial event, emphasizing the need for early diagnosis and intervention.

Physiologically, PE is defined primarily as a ventilation/perfusion (V/Q) abnormality in which areas of ventilated lung are not perfused. It is rare for this to be purely a perfusion defect. Incomplete redistribution of regional blood flow without changes in ventilation, right-to-left shunting of deoxygenated blood, resistance-induced decreases in regional capillary transit time, increased oxygen extraction (secondary to decreased cardiac output), and release of vasoactive mediators from platelets within thrombi and damaged endothelium, each contribute to the varying degrees of shunt and V/Q mismatch that underlie the broad spectrum of clinical presentation. Small emboli that pass through the pulmonary vasculature and lodge in the periphery of the lung are often asymptomatic. The more classic symptoms of pleuritic chest pain, hemoptysis, and dyspnea are only observed when emboli are associated with pulmonary infarction. Moderate-sized emboli, trapped in proximal segmental pulmonary vasculature, are associated with more severe dyspnea and hypoxemia. Larger emboli obstructing the pulmonary outflow tract are responsible for hemodynamic instability and sudden death.

Although hypoxemia, respiratory alkalosis, and tachycardia are common features and trigger the clinical suspicion of pulmonary embolism, these characteristics are neither universal nor specific. Infectious diseases, cardiogenic and noncardiogenic pulmonary edema, traumatic lung injuries, and other forms of respiratory distress, are often associated with a similar constellation of symptoms. On the other hand, while the degree of hypoxemia does correlate with the severity of the clinical PE syndrome, a normal A-a gradient and a normal $PaCO_2$ in a patient breathing room air are insufficient evidence to *rule out* the diagnosis. As many as 10% of patients with documented PE may have normal findings on measurement of blood gases. The spectrum of clinical presentation emphasizes the need for sensitive and specific means of distinguishing pulmonary embolism from other etiologies of respiratory distress.

Risk stratification for individual patients is a critical component to the development of a cost-effective diagnostic and management strategy. Well-recognized independent risk factors for development of DVT and subsequent PE include a history of previous DVT, older age, obesity, malignancy, inherited or acquired hypercoagulability states, recent trauma, and immobility (Table 10.1). These same risk factors also have a cumulative effect on the risk of DVT/PE. Geerts used a prospective cohort design to stratify surgical patients for their risk of DVT/PE based on age, presence of major or minor risk factors, and clinical setting (Table 10.2). This formula for assessment of risk can be particularly helpful for surgical patients in the perioperative period. Outside the perioperative period, a validated clinical decision tree, such as the Wells Criteria for Assessment of

TABLE 10.1. Major general risk factors for venous thromboembolism (VTE) (Reprinted from Geerts et al., 2004. With permission).

Surgery

Trauma

Immobility, paresis

Malignancy

Cancer therapy

Previous VTE

Increasing age

Pregnancy and postpartum period

Estrogen-containing contraceptives or hormonal replacement therapy

Selective estrogen receptor modulators

Acute medical illness

Heart or respiratory failure

Inflammatory bowel disease

Nephrotic syndrome

Myeloproliferative disease

Paroxysmal nocturnal hemoglobinuria

Obesity

Smoking

Varicose veins

Central venous catheterization

Inherited or acquired hypercoagulability

Pre-test Probability of Pulmonary Embolism (> Table 10.3), offers an objective way to stratify risk. A point-scoring method correlates data from the history and physical with the probability of PE for any individual patient. Once the risk of PE is calculated, this pre-test probability guides the subsequent work-up and leads to a post-test probability if the diagnosis is not definitive.

TABLE 10.2. Stratification of surgical patients according to VTE risk without prophylaxis (Reprinted from Geerts et al., 2004. With permission).

Category	Definition	Calf DVT (%)	Proximal DVT (%)	Clinical PE (%)	Fatal PE (%)
Low risk	Age <40 years, no risk factor, minor surgery	2	0.4	0.2	<0.01
Moderate risk	Presence of only one of the following:	10–20	2–4	1–2	0.1–0.4
	Age 40–60 years				
	Major surgery				
	Risk factor present				
High risk	Age > 60 years	20–40	4–8	2–4	0.4–1.0
	Age > 40 years + major surgery + risk factor present				
Highest risk	Age > 40 years + major surgery and:	40–80	10–20	4–10	0.2–5
	Previous VTE, cancer, or hypercoagulable condition				
	Major trauma				
	Spinal cord injury				
	Hip/knee arthroplasty				
	Hip surgery				

DVT, deep vein thrombosis; PE, pulmonary embolism; VTE, venous thromboembolism.

TABLE 10.3. Wells criteria for assessment of pre-test probability of pulmonary embolism (Data from Wells et al., 2000).

Criteria	Points
1. Suspected PE	3.0
2. An alternative diagnosis is less likely than PE	3.0
3. Heart rate > 100 beats/min	1.5
4. Immobilization or surgery in previous 4 weeks	1.5
5. Previous DVT/PE	1.5
6. Hemoptysis	1.0
7. Malignancy (on treatment or treated within past 6 months)	1.0

Score	Mean probability of PE	% of Patients with this score	Risk
<2	3.6	40	low
2–6	20.50%	53	medium
>6	66.70%	7	high

Diagnostic Tools

While an integral part of the assessment of respiratory distress, chest radiography is usually of little value in confirming the presence of PE. Increased lucency of a lung field (due to occlusion of the central pulmonary artery), atelectasis, small pleural effusions, or pleural-based wedge defects secondary to pulmonary infarctions are considered to be classic radiographic abnormalities, but they are absent in the majority of patients. As many as 40% of patients with PE have a normal study. The primary value of chest radiography is to rule out other etiologies of pulmonary dysfunction and to provide correlation for matching defects identified on V/Q scan.

Pulmonary angiography used to be the reference standard for the diagnosis of PE. Due to a small but significant rate of complications, as well as limited availability in many communities, pulmonary angiography has largely been supplanted by spiral CT angiogram of the chest (CTA). Recent studies confirm that the CTA is a cost-effective diagnostic modality with sensitivity and specificity rates of 90% and 94%, respectively, compared to conventional angiogram. For patients who have a contraindication for CT (e.g., contrast allergy or pregnancy), ventilation-perfusion scanning remains the generally accepted initial procedure of choice. Areas of mismatch, characterized by an absence of perfusion in the presence of normal ventilation, suggest PE. Areas of matching ventilation and perfusion deficits are more consistent with intrinsic lung disease. The sensitivity and specificity of V/Q scanning are such that a high probability scan coupled with a high pre-test risk probability yields a true positive diagnosis in 85–96% of cases. Fewer than 5% of patients for whom there is a low clinical suspicion of PE and a low probability scan are ultimately determined to have a thromboembolism and therefore may be safely managed without anticoagulation. The large percentage of patients with suspected PE and indeterminate probability scan, however, remain problematic. Further work-up, guided by their risk stratification and pre-test probability, should precede initiation of therapy.

Diagnostic Strategies

Several decision-analysis strategies combining noninvasive studies have been proposed to maximize diagnostic acumen if a definitive study such as CTA is not available. When the clinical presentation, chest radiography, and V/Q scanning suggest an intermediate probability of PE, Doppler examination of the upper or lower extremities can help to "rule in" the diagnosis of PE, if the presence of a DVT is accepted as an accurate surrogate to confirm the diagnosis of PE. Although the sensitivity of color Doppler ultrasonography in symptomatic patients has been reported to be as high as 98%, diagnosis of asymptomatic venous thrombosis, even in high-risk patients, has shown a disappointingly high degree of variability, ranging from 38% to 83%. In addition, since 56–67% of patients with angiographic evidence of PE also have negative lower extremity Doppler ultrasonographic examinations, the absence of ultrasonic evidence of DVT does not eliminate the possibility that PE has already occurred. Contrast-enhanced venography, impedance plethysmography, and radioisotope techniques have not been widely adopted in clinical practice owing to limitations in availability and sensitivity.

Another decision-analysis strategy, which has been tested in critically ill, ventilated patients at risk for a variety of respiratory complications, incorporates additional physiologic alterations associated with PE into the overall assessment of clinical probability. Since pulmonary emboli result in obstruction of perfusion without a change in airway patency, physiologic dead space is typically increased with significant thromboembolism. Physiologic dead space may be calculated by measuring end-tidal carbon dioxide. An abnormal result is typically considered to be >20% and is consistent with, though not diagnostic of, PE. D-dimer is a fibrin degradation product formed by the enzymatic activity of cross-linked fibrin polymers. Although always present in patients with thromboembolic states, D-dimer can also be detected in other physiologic states, such as malignancy, post-injury, and pregnancy. A negative D-dimer assay, therefore, can safely rule out the diagnosis of PE in patients with a low pre-test probability, but a positive assay necessitates further testing. Although neither calculation of a high physiologic dead space nor a positive D-dimer test is specific to the diagnosis of PE, their combination does provide some predictive value in that a normal D-dimer and alveolar-dead space percentage carries a false-negative rate of <1%. The positive predictive value of these tests, however, is less certain.

Treatment Strategies

For the majority of patients, anticoagulation with unfractionated heparin remains the therapeutic mainstay for pulmonary embolism. In addition to minimizing the recurrence of PE, anticoagulation limits the long-term sequelae of lower extremity venous stasis associated with an underlying phlebitic obstruction.

The immediate goal is to prevent further clot formation. Clot dissolution proceeds through venous fibrinolysis and is largely unaffected by heparin. Therapeutic anticoagulation, as measured by an activated partial thromboplastin time (PTT) of 1.5–2.5 times control values, should be achieved as rapidly as possible since mortality increases in direct proportion to delays in treatment. Patients with excessive levels of heparin-binding proteins will require more than the typical loading dose of 100–200 U/kg, followed by continuous 30,000 U per 24 h infusion of unfractionated heparin to achieve effective anticoagulation. Side effects of heparin include bleeding, hyperkalemia, and thrombocytopenia. Heparin-induced thrombocytopenia and the associated thrombosis syndrome occur in approximately 3% of patients treated with unfractionated heparin and are the result of antibodies to heparin-platelet factor 4 complexes.

In light of these potential complications and following successful trials demonstrating efficacy in DVT prophylaxis, low molecular weight heparins (LMWHs) have been proposed as therapeutic alternatives to unfractionated heparin for the treatment of PE. To date, investigations comparing LMWH to intravenous heparin have shown similar PE recurrence rates, mortality, and bleeding complications. Because these drugs have longer half-lives, LMWHs do offer the benefit of single dose, subcutaneous administration without the need for vigilant monitoring of clotting times. As a result, patients can be treated as an outpatient with LMWHs while awaiting therapeutic anticoagulation with warfarin. However, LMWHs are more difficult to reverse than unfractionated heparin, which poses a potentially significant problem should bleeding complications occur, especially in a post-surgical or post-trauma patient. Conversion to oral warfarin should be started within 3 days of beginning heparin. A transient hypercoagulable state is paradoxically associated with the initiation of warfarin; thus, treatment should overlap intravenous therapy until the international normalized ratio (INR) stabilizes in the therapeutic range (2–3) for at least 48 h.

The choice of initial treatment depends on the severity of physiologic compromise. For patients with hemodynamic

instability, right-heart failure secondary to massive thromboembolism in the pulmonary outflow tract is usually fatal
unless aggressive interventions to relieve the acute obstruction
can be employed. In patients for whom there is a high suspicion and probability of PE and no contraindication to therapy,
initiation of anticoagulation before imaging studies to confirm
the diagnosis should be strongly considered. Supplemental
oxygen, mechanical ventilation, invasive hemodynamic monitoring, and inotropic support all have a place in management.
If there is no compelling contraindication, early thrombolysis
is recommended, as there is clear evidence of improved mortality rates in patients with hemodynamic instability due to PE.
Thrombolysis with streptokinase, urokinase, or recombinant
tissue-type plasminogen activator (rt-PA) has been advocated
as a means of relieving acute pulmonary hypertension and
right-heart failure. Unlike heparin, thrombolytics are also
effective for the dissolution of established thrombi, and thus
may also be useful in the management of patients who present
late in their clinical course (up to 14 days after PE).

Debate remains as to the most effective thrombolytic agent.
Confounding variables include allergic reactions to streptokinase and urokinase, local versus systemic administration, and
the relative balance of clot resolution with the frequency of
bleeding complications. While directed thrombolysis offers an
effective means for improving pulmonary outflow, the unavoidable systemic effects of clot dissolution pose a significant relative contraindication to its use in the post-trauma or post-surgical
patient with coincident massive PE. Surgical embolectomy
(Trendelenburg procedure) and catheter embolectomy are
safe alternatives in these hemodynamically unstable patients
for whom thrombolytic therapy presents an equally life-threatening, potential risk of bleeding. Surgical pulmonary embolectomy may be life-saving, but it is not readily available in most
centers. Transvenous catheter pulmonary embolectomy, on the
other hand, can be performed in conjunction with diagnostic
pulmonary arteriography, avoiding median sternotomy and the
potential need for cardiopulmonary bypass. Massive thrombi
may be disrupted or extracted (aspirated) in as many as 76%
of cases with significant reductions in pulmonary artery

pressure and improvement in cardiac function. Treatment should be followed by anticoagulation with standard unfractionated heparin or warfarin therapy. To date, no formal clinical trials comparing directed thrombolysis with embolectomy have been conducted. However, nonrandomized trials comparing catheter embolectomy and heparin to surgical embolectomy and vena cava clipping show similar survival rates.

The placement of a vena cava filter is an appropriate alternative in hemodynamically stable patients with an absolute contradiction to anticoagulant therapy (e.g., head trauma), complications requiring cessation of anticoagulation, or recurrent embolism in the setting of appropriate therapy. In recent years, the use of temporary, retrievable filters have grown in use and are attractive as a "bridge to therapy" when the clinical condition may permit eventual anticoagulation.

Outcomes

Resolution of DVT and respiratory compromise associated with primary and recurrent PE depends on the clinical treatment strategy. Although recanalization occurs in 99% of leg vein segments after anticoagulation therapy, a single episode of DVT increases the risk of developing chronic lower extremity valvular incompetence by a factor of 10. The postphlebitic syndrome, characterized by stasis ulcerations and limitations to ambulation, carries the added personal and economic costs of poor wound healing and limitations to activity with secondary work restrictions.

The duration of warfarin anticoagulation to treat DVT complicated by PE is the subject of ongoing debate. Indeed, the duration of therapy is dependent on a patient's underlying risk factors for developing DVT and whether these risk factors are temporary (e.g., post-surgical), permanent (e.g., in the setting of coagulation disorders), or idiopathic. The risks of bleeding should also be considered for patients who need long-term or lifelong anticoagulation. Three months of anticoagulation is usually adequate for patients who have an identifiable and temporary risk factor for DVT; the recurrence rate in this population is low. Recommendations for patients with underlying coagulation disorders have not been established with clinical trials. However, patients with an associated malignancy; factor V Leiden defect; deficiencies of plasminogen, plasminogen activator, anti-thrombin III, or protein C or S; myeloproliferative disorders, including polycythemia vera; systemic lupus erythematosus; homocystinuria; and those with "idiopathic" causes for DVT, should probably remain on anticoagulants for at least 6 months, if not indefinitely, after a single episode of venous thrombosis.

A small percentage of patients develop chronic thromboembolic pulmonary hypertension (CTEPH) after PE despite appropriate anticoagulation therapy. This frequently underdiagnosed syndrome is surgically correctable, but must be distinguished from primary pulmonary hypertension complicated by right-sided heart failure. These patients present with gradual onset of worsening exertional dyspnea, hypoxemia, and right-sided heart failure after an asymptomatic period. The early clues to the diagnosis include disproportionately severe symptoms that are unexplained by spirometric measurements and the presence of flow murmurs over the lung field. Pulmonary and hemodynamic signs and symptoms progress without evidence of new perfusion defects on serial V/Q scans, suggesting the involvement of smaller, peripheral pulmonary vessels in the presence of a partially recanalized, proximal pulmonary vasculature. A modest degree of resting pulmonary hypertension, which may be demonstrated with echocardiography, is markedly worsened by exercise. Right-sided heart catheterization in addition to pulmonary angiography is essential to quantify the degree of pulmonary hypertension, rule out competing diagnoses, and define the surgical accessibility of the obstructing thrombotic lesions. This procedure should be delayed for several months after an acute embolic event to allow for maximal resolution and organization of the embolus and avoid an interruption of anticoagulant therapy. Regardless of whether surgical intervention is entertained, patients with demonstrated CTEPH should receive lifelong anticoagulation with a goal INR between 2 and 3.

Surgical treatment of chronic pulmonary thromboembolism is appropriate for symptomatic patients but requires a multidisciplinary approach for diagnosis and management. Careful selection, especially with respect to comorbidities, is mandatory because of the procedural morbidity and mortality, as well as the observation that not all patients with CTEPH benefit from surgery. For those patients not considered surgical candidates, treatment with sildenafil (phosphodiesterase-5 inhibitor) and bosentan (endothelin receptor antagonist) have shown promising preliminary results but have yet to be tested in controlled trials.

Prevention

Clearly, if improved clinical outcomes are to be realized and the complications of PE avoided, practitioners should focus on prevention. The high incidence and potentially devastating consequences of venous thromboembolism mandate the use of DVT prophylaxis in patients at risk. Well-controlled clinical trials have documented the positive impact of prophylactic pharmacologic regimens and intermittent pneumatic compression devices in patients with two or more significant risk factors. Despite wide acceptance of these data, preventive measures are often omitted from routine medical practice.

In addition to serving as a guide to diagnostic testing, assessment of clinical risk is crucial to appropriate prevention strategies. The majority of controlled trials delineating the risk of thromboembolism have focused on surgical patients. Available data, however, suggest that relative risk reductions in the incidence of DVT are comparable between medical and surgical patients. The risk stratification scheme proposed by Geerts offers prophylaxis guidelines based on risk. These guidelines are recommended by the American College of Chest Physicians and were developed after extensive review of the literature and expert consensus (Table 10.4).

Many studies have proposed the use of vena cava filters as primary prophylaxis in certain patient populations. Studies assessing the long-term effects of permanent vena cava filters

TABLE 10.4. Guidelines for prophylaxis of venous thromboembolism in surgical patients according to risk category (Data from Geerts et al., 2004).

Category	Definition	Prevention strategy
Low risk	Age < 40 years, no RF, minor surgery	Aggressive and early mobilization
Moderate risk	Presence of only one of the following: Age 40–60 years Major surgery RF present	LDUH every 12 h, LMWH, or GCS/IPC (if bleeding risk)
High risk	Age > 60 years Age > 40 + major surgery + RF present	LDUH every 8 h, LMWH, or IPC (if bleeding risk)
Highest risk	Age > 40 + major surgery and: Previous VTE, cancer, or hypercoagulable condition Major trauma Spinal cord injury Hip/knee arthroplasty Hip surgery	LMWH (trauma, spinal cord injury) LDUH every 8 h + GCS/IPC or LMWH + GCS/IPC Consider extended prophylaxis for cancer or spinal cord injury

GCS, graduated compression stockings; IPC, intermittent pneumatic compression; LDUH, low-dose unfractionated heparin; LMWH, low-molecular weight heparin; VTE, venous thromboembolism, RF, Risk factor.

have demonstrated a decreased risk of PE but no difference in mortality and an increase in the risk of recurrent DVT. The use of retrievable filters is an attractive option in those patients where the contraindication to anticoagulation is thought to be temporary. After filter removal, these patients need anticoagulation for only a defined period of time and thus avoid the long-term complications of a permanent filter and prolonged anticoagulation. However, reports vary widely (15–87%) as to the actual rate of successful retrieval of these temporary filters. Furthermore, since most retrievable filters are relatively new, there are no data as to their long-term performance if they are not retrieved.

Selected Readings

Ansell J (2005) Vena cava filters: do we know all that we need to know? Circulation 112:298–299

Geerts WH, Pineo GF, Heit JA, et al. (2004) Prevention of venous thromboembolism: the Seventh ACCP Conference on Antithrombotic and Thrombolytic Therapy. Chest 126(Suppl 3): 338S–400S. Review

Hoeper MM, Mayer E, Simonneau G, et al. (2006) Chronic thromboembolic pulmonary hypertension. Circulation 113:2011–2020. Review

Jerges-Sanches C, Ramirez-Rivera A, de Lourdes Garcia M, et al. (1995) Streptokinase and heparin versus heparin alone in massive pulmonary embolism: a randomized controlled trial. J Thromb Thrombolysis 2:227–229

Kline JA, Israel EG, Michelson EA, et al. (2001) Diagnostic accuracy of a bedside D-dimer assay and alveolar dead-space measurement for rapid exclusion of pulmonary embolism: a multicenter study. JAMA 285:761–768

Legere B, Dweik R, Arroliga A (1999) Venous thromboembolism in the intensive care unit. Clin Chest Med 20:367–384, ix. Review

Perrier A, Bounameaux H, Morabia A, et al. (1996) Diagnosis of pulmonary embolism by a decision analysis-based strategy including clinical probability, D-dimer levels, and ultrasonography: a management study. Arch Intern Med 156:531–536

Qanadli SD, Hajjam ME, Mesurolle B, et al. (2000) Pulmonary embolism detection: prospective evaluation of dual-section helical CT versus selective pulmonary arteriography in 157 patients. Radiology 217:447–455

van Erkel AR, van Rossum AB, Bloem JL, et al. (1996) Spiral CT angiography for suspected pulmonary embolism: a cost-effectiveness analysis. Radiology 201:29–36

Wells PS, Anderson DR, Ginsberg J (2000) Assessment of deep vein thrombosis or pulmonary embolism by the combined use of clinical model and noninvasive diagnostic tests. Semin Thromb Hemost 26:643–656. Review

Wells PS, Anderson DR, Rodger M, et al. (2000) Derivation of a simple clinical model to categorize patients probability of pulmonary embolism: increasing the models utility with the SimpliRED D-dimer. Thromb Haemost 83:416–420

11
Right Ventricular Failure and Cardiogenic Shock

James K. Kirklin and Ayesha S. Bryant

Pearls and Pitfalls

- The most common presentation of acute right ventricular failure includes in the setting of inferior myocardial infarction, usually following acute proximal occlusion of a dominant right coronary artery.
- A key modality for diagnosis of isolated right ventricular failure includes transthoracic echocardiography.
- In the presence of acute right ventricular failure, invasive hemodynamic monitoring with a pulmonary artery catheter facilitates diagnostic and therapeutic decisions.
- Initial therapy of right ventricular failure includes inotropic support (usually with milrinone or dobutamine) and administration of colloid or crystallized solutions to a targeted central venous pressure of 18–22 mmHg in order to provide adequate left ventricular filling.
- The administration of agents such as nitric oxide which directly reduce pulmonary vascular resistance is a key component of therapy for right ventricular failure.
- Cardiogenic shock is the leading cause of in-hospital mortality following acute myocardial infarction.
- Despite recent advancements in therapy, hospital mortality approaches 50% when acute myocardial infarction is complicated by cardiogenic shock.

K.I. Bland et al. (eds.), *Critical Care Surgery*,
DOI 10.1007/978-1-84996-378-7_11,
© Springer-Verlag London Limited 2011

- In profound shock, compensatory mechanisms to support cardiac output such as sympathetic stimulation and peripheral vasoconstriction become maladaptive and contribute to mortality.
- Cardiogenic shock is accompanied by a systemic inflammatory response that potentiates end organ damage.
- Once the clinical syndrome of shock is identified, transthoracic echocardiographic evaluation is essential for identification of a cardiac etiology.
- The current ACC/AHA recommendations for acute MI complicated by cardiogenic shock include early invasive reperfusion for patients less than 75 years of age.
- Intra-aortic balloon pump support and/or mechanical circulatory support should be considered for stabilization of deteriorating hemodynamics and preservation of end-organ function in the presence of cardiogenic shock.
- Despite the high hospital mortality, survivors of myocardial infarction complicated by shock have a favorable long-term outcome.

Right Ventricular Failure

Introduction

Right ventricular failure forms an important subset of congestive heart failure, which affects more than 4.5 million Americans, with over 500,000 new cases diagnosed each year. More prevalent in the elderly, this condition affects approximately 10% of patients over 75 years of age. Furthermore, congestive heart failure is the leading hospital discharge diagnosis in individuals over age 65 years. The pathophysiology of and clinical conditions leading to heart failure provides insights into unique differences between the right and left ventricles, both in normal as well as pathological states.

Pathophysiology of Right Ventricular Failure

The right ventricle consists of two anatomically and functionally distinct cavities (the sinus portion and the outlet chamber or infundibulum). During right ventricular contraction, pressure is generated in the sinus portion with a systolic motion beginning at the apex and moving towards the infundibulum. Due to the compliance of the infundibulum and the relatively thin walled right ventricle, the peak pressure is reduced and prolonged. The right ventricle normally has sustained ejection during pressure development, and this prolonged low-pressure emptying makes the right ventricle very sensitive to changes in afterload. During states of chronically increased afterload, the right ventricle compensates by dilating to maintain stroke volume, though the ejection fraction is reduced and the synchronized contraction of right ventricular components is lost. With increased afterload, the isovolumic contraction phase and ejection time are prolonged, which increases myocardial oxygen consumption.

The right ventricle is primarily perfused by the right coronary artery, with the supply of some regions via the left anterior descending artery. In contrast to left ventricular perfusion, which continues predominantly during diastole, right coronary artery blood flow continues during both systole and diastole. In the presence of important pulmonary artery hypertension, the coronary perfusion gradient is less favorable during systole, and right coronary artery flow occurs mainly during diastole, reducing oxygen supply in the presence of increased demand.

Both the right ventricular free wall (supplied by the right coronary artery) and the interventricular septum (supplied by the posterior descending artery and branches of the left anterior descending artery) importantly contribute to right ventricular contraction. Thus, decreases in perfusion pressure to the right coronary artery have an important adverse affect on free wall contraction, and left ventricular dysfunction involving the interventricular septum adversely affects the septal contribution to right ventricular function.

A major contributor to the clinical sequelae of right ventricular failure is tricuspid regurgitation, which is a common component of the failing right ventricle. The tricuspid valve is anatomically more vulnerable to regurgitation induced by ventricular dilatation than the systemic mitral valve, since the tricuspid valve is crescentic in shape (unlike the circular mitral orifice) and the papillary muscles of the right ventricle are multiple and small (compared to the two large papillary muscles of the mitral valve).

Right ventricular ejection fraction is determined by intrinsic right ventricular contractile function and by right ventricular preload and afterload. The deleterious effects of functional derangements of one ventricle on the performance of the other is termed **ventricular interdependence**. Thus, left ventricular failure, with the resultant increase in pulmonary capillary wedge pressure and pulmonary artery pressure, increases right ventricular afterload and subsequent right ventricular dysfunction. When right ventricular end diastolic volume is increased secondary to chronic increases in right ventricular afterload, the resultant shift of the interventricular septum towards the left ventricular cavity during diastole (contributed to in part by the restrictive effect of the pericardium on the right ventricular free wall) results in impairment of left ventricular filling. Septal displacement of the failing left ventricle increases right ventricular end diastolic pressure, promotes right ventricular dilatation, and increases the tendency for tricuspid regurgitation.

Clinical Presentation of Right Ventricular Failure

Right ventricular failure can present either acutely or as a chronic manifestation of heart failure. The most common presentation of acute right ventricular failure is in the setting of **inferior myocardial infarction**. The typical situation is acute proximal occlusion of a dominant right coronary artery resulting in extensive right ventricular infarction. When the left coronary circulation is dominant (posterior descending artery arising from the distal circumflex), acute occlusion of the left circumflex coronary artery may result in right ventricular infarction. Marked reduction in right ventricular systolic function with inadequate left ventricular filling produces low cardiac output and hypotension, while the alterations in right ventricular compliance promote increased right atrial and central venous pressure.

Acute right ventricular failure/dysfunction is an important complication following certain **cardiac operations**, in particular cardiac transplantation, mitral valve disease with pulmonary hypertension, certain forms of congenital heart disease, and ischemic heart disease. The transplanted right ventricle is very sensitive to increased afterload, and the right ventricle is more susceptible than the left ventricle to inadequate myocardial preservation, particularly in the setting of moderate or marked increases in post transplant vascular resistance. In operations for congenital heart disease, such as in repair of tetralogy of Fallot, direct surgical procedures on or within the right ventricle predispose to right ventricular dysfunction secondary to myocardial injury or creation of pulmonary insufficiency by placement of a transannular patch when there is important obstruction at the level of the pulmonary annulus. In the setting of ischemic heart disease or mitral valve disease with pulmonary hypertension, the presence of important left ventricular dysfunction following operation (with the accompanying marked elevation of left atrial pressure) can induce severe pulmonary hypertension in a reactive pulmonary vasculature. Right ventricular failure may ensue, particularly if the right ventricle is already compromised.

Right ventricular failure secondary to **chronic pulmonary hypertension** (whether the primary etiology is chronic left ventricular failure, chronic lung disease, primary pulmonary hypertension, or pulmonary thromboembolic disease) results from chronic pressure overload and associated volume overload when tricuspid regurgitation becomes severe. In this setting, ascites and lower extremity edema may accompany signs and symptoms of low cardiac output.

Diagnosis

The major modality for diagnosis of right ventricular failure is transthoracic echocardiography. Typical findings include marked depression of right ventricular systolic function, dilatation of the right ventricle, and frequently, moderate to severe tricuspid insufficiency. The echocardiogram provides useful information to distinguish right ventricular dysfunction from other conditions which can induce marked right atrial hypertension including constrictive pericarditis, pericardial effusion with tamponade, and severe tricuspid stenosis.

In the presence of true acute right ventricular failure (as opposed to dysfunction), invasive hemodynamic monitoring with a pulmonary artery catheter capable of measuring thermodilution cardiac output greatly facilitates diagnostic and therapeutic decisions. Whether right ventricular failure occurs secondary to acute myocardial infarction, following cardiac surgery, or from other causes, the hallmark of isolated right ventricular failure is the marked discrepancy between right atrial (or central venous) pressure and pulmonary capillary wedge (or left atrial) pressure. Right atrial pressure is nearly always greater than 15 mmHg in the presence of a normal left atrial or capillary wedge pressure (12 mmHg or less). Depending on the severity of right ventricular failure, cardiac index is reduced (usually 2.0 l/min/m^2 or less). The presence or absence of pulmonary artery hypertension critically influences the selection of therapeutic modalities for augmentation of right ventricular function.

Treatment

Therapy for right ventricular failure focuses on treatment of the underlying etiology if specific therapy is available (such as in treatment of acute myocardial infarction) plus interventions directed at preload adjustment, augmentation of right ventricular contractility, and reduction of right ventricular afterload.

Augmentation of Preload

Volume administration is required when right ventricular failure is severe enough that left ventricular filling is inadequate to generate sufficient cardiac output for adequate organ perfusion. This frequently involves infusion of crystalloid or colloid solutions to a targeted central venous pressure of 18–22 mmHg. When right ventricular failure responds to augmentation of contractility or afterload reduction (see below), the lowest right atrial pressure consistent with adequate cardiac output is desirable. This underscores the importance of direct measurement of right atrial and pulmonary artery pressures as well as cardiac output during the first 48–72 h of therapy. Whole blood or packed red blood cells are initially infused to achieve a hematocrit of 36–40. Once the targeted hematocrit is achieved, additional infusions should consist of colloid (albumin or fresh frozen plasma), although compelling evidence is lacking for the superiority of colloid solutions over saline.

Drugs to Increase Contractility

The most desirable inotropes for right ventricular support are those which increase cardiac contractility, while at the same time reducing pulmonary vascular resistance. Milrinone, dobutamine, and isoproterenol produce a variable reduction in pulmonary vascular resistance and are the most commonly employed inotropic agents for right ventricular failure in the presence of normal or nearly normal systemic blood pressure. Milrinone differs from sympathomimetic agents in that it is in the class of phosphodiesterase inhibitors, which do not act through direct stimulation of adrenergic receptors. Instead, their inotropic effects are exerted through inhibition of phosphodiesterase F-3 (a membrane-based enzyme responsible for the breakdown of cyclic-AMP), resulting in increases in calcium influx. In the presence of systemic hypotension combined with right ventricular failure, combination inotropic therapy is often advisable, with agents such as dopamine and milrinone or dopamine and dobutamine. The recommended dosages of various inotropic agents are discussed in the section on *Treatment of Cardiogenic Shock*.

In the presence of systemic hypotension, vasopressin is a particularly effective agent in that it increases systemic blood pressure, and thereby, may indirectly increase right ventricular perfusion and right ventricular contractility even though it does not have direct positive inotropic effects itself. In addition, vasopressin has a direct pulmonary vasodilator effects. When administered in doses of 0.01 – 0.04 units/kg/min, vasopressin increases systemic vascular resistance while potentially dilating the coronary and pulmonary arterial circulation.

Reduction of Right Ventricular Afterload

As noted in the previous section, inotropic agents such as milrinone, isoproterenol (Table 11.1), and dobutamine, as well as vasopressin may directly reduce pulmonary vascular resistance. Although a number of direct pulmonary vasodilating agents (without inotropic effects) have been utilized in

TABLE 11.1. Properties of vasodilator agents (Adapted from Kirklin et al., 2004).

	Systemic arterial vasodilation	Pulmonary arterial vasodilation	Positive inotropic effect	Increase in systemic venous capacitance
Isoproterenol	++	+++	++++	0
Milrinone	+++	+++	+++	0
Nitroprusside	++++	+++	0	0
Nitroglycerin	++	++	0	+++
Prostaglandin E1	+++	+++	0	0
Prostacyclin	++	+++	0	0
Nitric oxide	0	+++++	0	0

the past, these have been largely supplanted by inhaled nitric oxide, which has profound pulmonary vasodilator effects. Inhaled nitric oxide can be administered via an endotracheal tube when the patient is mechanically ventilated or via face mask administration. Nitric oxide is generally initiated at 20–40 parts per million in the presence of pulmonary hypertension. When right ventricular function improves and a target pulmonary artery pressure of 35–40 mmHg systolic pressure is achieved, gradual tapering of nitric oxide is initiated. When nitric oxide is reduced to less than about 10 parts per million, very slow weaning should be accomplished because of the potential for rebound pulmonary hypertension following abrupt nitric oxide withdrawal. Recently, inhaled prostacyclin has proved useful in the treatment of right heart failure following cardiac surgery.

In the presence of coexisting severe left ventricular dysfunction and elevated left atrial pressure (particularly in the setting of myocardial ischemia), intravenous nitroglycerin (dose 0.5–2 µg/kg/min) is a useful agent to lower left atrial pressure (via a direct coronary vasodilator effect and through increasing systemic venous capacitance) and secondarily neutralize reactive pulmonary hypertension.

Additional Therapeutic Strategies

In the setting of acute inferior myocardial infarction secondary to right coronary artery or circumflex occlusion, **emergent revascularization** with thrombolytic agents, angioplasty, or surgical revascularization is advisable. Since approximately one-half of overall right ventricular function is derived from the right ventricular free wall and half from the intraventricular septum, revascularization of these areas may include consideration of right ventricular marginal arteries in the revascularization plan.

In the presence of decompensated heart failure secondary to progressive right ventricular dysfunction, administration of **nesiritide**, a synthetic form of B-type (brain) natriuretic peptide, may facilitate fluid removal when other diuretics have been unsuccessful. This hormone increases sodium and water excretion and decreases renin and aldosterone secretion without activation of the sympathetic nervous system, thus promoting reduction in preload, pulmonary artery pressure, right atrial pressure and systemic vascular resistance. Nesiritide is usually combined with loop diuretic therapy using a planned continuous infusion for 2–3 days. The generally recommended dose includes a 0.3 µg bolus followed by an infusion of 0.015–0.03 µg/kg/min.

When the measures noted above are inadequate in providing effective systemic perfusion, consideration should be given to **mechanical circulatory support** of the right ventricle. The **Abiomed BVS 5000** (Danvers, Mass) is a short term (1–4 weeks) extracorporeal pulsatile pump that can be used for right, left, or biventricular support. The **Thoratec** (Pleasanton, CA) pneumatic paracorporeal ventricular assist device is a longer-term ventricular assist device which has been utilized for right-, left-, or bi-ventricular support in the United States for over 20 years. Anticoagulation with Warfarin and antiplatelet agents is necessary for prevention of thromboembolism. For smaller patients, the Berlin Heart (Berlin, Germany) (approved in Europe but not yet FDA-approved in the United States) provides similar univentricular or biventricular support with a variety of pump sizes down to 10 ml (for infants) (Fig. 11.1).

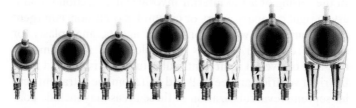

FIGURE 11.1. The Berlin Heart paracorporeal ventricular assist device is available in a range of pump sizes from 10 to 80 ml (Courtesy of Berlin Heart AG, Berlin, Germany) (Reprinted from International Heart and Lung Transplantation Monograph Series, vol. 1: mechanical circulatory support, copyright 2006. With permission from the International Society for Heart and Lung Transplantation).

More recently, percutaneous technology that can be applied in the cath lab includes right ventricular support with the Tandem heart (Pittsburgh, PA), which withdraws blood from the right atrium and infuses it directly into the pulmonary artery.

Outcomes

In patients with chronic heart failure the presence of severe right ventricular dysfunction is a powerful predictor of mortality in both dilated cardiomyopathy and in ischemic heart disease. Acute right ventricular failure in the setting of inferior myocardial infarction is associated with approximately a threefold increase in hospital mortality. A dramatic reduction in hospital mortality has been documented with successful primary angioplasty of the coronary vessel causing right ventricular compromise. When acute right ventricular failure complicates cardiac operations, the prognosis is generally favorable when left ventricular function is good and effective cardiac output is restored at a right atrial pressure less than 20 mmHg (without mechanical support) within about 48 h.

Cardiogenic Shock

Introduction

Cardiogenic shock may be defined as inadequate perfusion of the microcirculation to sustain viability of vital organs secondary to a primary cardiac etiology which, if uncorrected, results in death. Cardiogenic shock due to primary pump failure is the leading cause of in-hospital mortality following acute myocardial infarction. Despite numerous advances in the care of patients with myocardial infarction including early revascularization, the mortality remains high, in the range of 50–80% depending upon the specific patient risk profile. With improved understanding of the potential reversibility of stunned or hibernating myocardium following restoration of blood flow, there is a current major emphasis on prompt revascularization. Survivability of cardiogenic shock from other etiologies depends on prompt inotropic and/or mechanical circulatory support of the failing heart.

Pathophysiology

The brain and heart are the two human organs with an absolute aerobic requirement. In an adult at rest, the coronary circulation supplies about 70–80 ml blood/100 g of myocardial tissue/min, from which the myocardium extracts 8–10 ml of O_2/100 g/min. Thus, myocardial mitochondria generate enormous quantities of ATP to meet the cellular ATP demand. During anaerobic metabolism secondary to acute coronary artery occlusion, inadequate ATP generation for surface membrane ion pumps results in marked cellular swelling, which if progressive causes cell death.

In the absence of a mechanical complication of myocardial infarction (such as papillary muscle rupture, ventricular septal defect, or ventricular rupture), an estimated 40% loss of left ventricular myocardium due to severe ischemia or necrosis is required to produce sufficient reduction in stroke volume (and overall cardiac output) to induce cardiogenic shock. Areas of ischemic but not infarcted myocardium are further compromised by the vicious cycle of decreased systolic and increased ventricular diastolic blood pressure, both of which reduce myocardial perfusion pressure (the gradient between coronary diastolic and left ventricular diastolic pressures). In the setting of markedly reduced coronary blood flow secondary to acute vessel occlusion, increasing diastolic pressures associated with pump failure act to increase wall stress, which elevates myocardial oxygen requirements and promotes further ischemia. The metabolic byproducts of reduced organ perfusion, such as lactic acidosis, further depress myocardial function. Compensatory mechanisms to support cardiac output, including sympathetic stimulation to increase heart rate and contractility, produce vasoconstriction which, when severe, reduces renal blood flow and increases left ventricular afterload. These compensatory mechanisms may eventually have a more deleterious than beneficial effect and become maladaptive, hastening the spiral toward death.

Another maladaptive response to the development of cardiogenic shock is a systemic inflammatory state which may potentiate end organ damage. Local tissue ischemia and necrosis stimulates the innate immune system, activating complement and leukocytes which increase local capillary permeability, resulting in further tissue damage. Nitric oxide (NO) likely augments the inflammatory response to cardiogenic shock. NO is normally synthesized by endothelial NO synthase and has cardioprotective effects at normal physiologic levels. Cardiogenic shock induces an upregulation of nitric oxide synthase, mediated by Interleukin-6 and possibly other cytokines. At high pathologic levels, NO suppresses mitochondrial respiration and reduces contractility in nonischemic myocardium. High NO levels also reduce the myocardial inotropic response to b-adrenergic stimulants and cause systemic vasodilation, further promoting the hypotensive state of shock.

Diagnosis

Various criteria have been used to describe the severity of cardiac derangement that constitutes shock. In general, systolic blood pressure is 90 or less in the absence of vasoactive drugs, cardiac index is less than 2.0 l/m/m^2, and there is clinical evidence of end-organ hypoperfusion as indicated by decreased urine output, cool and constricted extremities, and often depressed sensorium. The general clinical features that distinguish cardiac from non-cardiac causes of shock are listed in Table 11.2. Appropriate evaluation for acute myocardial infarction is of the greatest urgency, since emergent revascularization or correction of a mechanical complication

TABLE 11.2. Rapid formulation of a working diagnosis for the cause of shock (Reprinted from Holmes et al., 2003, copyright 2003. With permission from Elsevier).

Diagnostic issue	High-output hypotension: vasodilatory shock	Low cardiac-output hypotension: cardiogenic and hypovolemic shock
Is cardiac output reduced?	No	Yes
Pulse pressure	Wide	Narrow
Diastolic pressure	Extremely low	Low
Extremities, digits	Warm	Cool
Nailbed return	Rapid	Slow
Heart sounds	Crisp	Muffled
Temperature	Abnormally high or low	Normal
White blood cell count	Abnormally high or low	Normal
Site of infection	Present	Absent
	Reduced pump function: cardiogenic shock	Reduced venous return: hypovolemic shock
Is the heart too full?	Yes	No
Symptoms, clinical context	Angina, abnormal ECG	Blood loss, volume depletion
Jugular venous pressure	High	Low
Gallop rhythm	Present	Absent
Respiratory examinations	Crepitations	Normal
Chest radiograph	Large heart, pulmonary edema	Normal
What does not fit?		
Overlapping causes	High right atrial pressure hypotension	Nonresponsive hypovolemia

(continued)

TABLE 11.2. (continued)

Diagnostic issue	High-output hypotension: vasodilatory shock	Low cardiac-output hypotension: cardiogenic and hypovolemic shock
Septic cardiogenic	High right sided pressure, clear lungs	Adrenal insufficiency
Septic hypovolemic	Pulmonary embolus	Anaphylaxis
Cardiogenic hypovolemic	Right ventricular infarction	Neurogenic shock
	Cardiac tamponade	

TABLE 11.3. Causes of left ventricular dysfunction in the etiology of cardiogenic shock.

Systolic dysfunction

Myocardial infarction

Ischemia and global hypoxemia

Cardiomyopathy

Myocardial drugs

Beta-blocker overdose

Calcium channel blockers

Myocardial contusion

Respiratory acidosis

Metabolic derangements: acidosis, hypophosphatemia, hypocalcemia

Diastolic dysfunction

Ischemia and global hypoxemia

Ventricular hypertrophy

Restrictive cardiomyopathy

Ventricular interdependence

Greatly increased afterload

Critical aortic stenosis

Critical fixed or dynamic left ventricular outflow tract obstruction of myocardial infarction offers the best chance for survival. Other causes of cardiogenic shock are listed in Table 11.3. Transthoracic echocardiography is the best modality for the prompt diagnosis of mitral insufficiency or ruptured ventricular septum and assessment of the degree of depression of overall left and right ventricular systolic function. Accumulation of fluid or clot within the pericardial space suggests the possibility of ventricular rupture.

Hemodynamic monitoring with a Swan-Ganz catheter is necessary to quantify the severity of depressed cardiac output and the response to therapy. Large "V" waves on the capillary wedge tracing indicates severe mitral insufficiency and a step-up in oxygen saturation from the right atrium to the pulmonary artery suggests a ruptured interventricular septum. Prompt coronary angiography in the presence of acute myocardial infarction and shock offers the opportunity for prompt revascularization through either angioplasty or emergency surgery.

When cardiogenic shock develops in the absence of acute myocardial infarction, echocardiographic assessment is the cornerstone of diagnosis once the clinical syndrome is identified. Determination of the presence and the severity of ventricular dysfunction is often the most rapid method of distinguishing cardiogenic shock from non-cardiac causes.

Treatment

Initial Management

Initial management includes supplemental oxygen and rapid assessment of circulatory status. In the presence of depressed oxygen saturation despite supplemental oxygen (saturation less than about 90%), if increased work of breathing occurs, or if profound low cardiac output is present, intubation and mechanical ventilation is necessary. Correction of electrolyte abnormalities, detection and treatment of arrhythmias, and management of pain and anxiety should be implemented.

The importance of placement of a pulmonary artery catheter is underscored by the frequency of low pulmonary capillary wedge pressure in the face of low cardiac output, indicating the need for fluid administration while accurately monitoring pulmonary artery and central venous pressures.

Inotropic Support

Appropriate selection of inotropic support is a key component of therapy for cardiogenic shock. After initial support with dopamine, norepinephrine, or other alpha-adrenergic agents, refinement of inotropic support is directed by the circulatory state, measurements obtained from the pulmonary artery catheter, renal function (and urine output), right and left ventricular function, and the etiology of cardiogenic shock. The specification and doses of individual inotropes are listed in Tables 11.4 and 11.5.

Emergent Revascularization after Acute Myocardial Infarction

Percutaneous angioplasty and stenting of the infarct-related vessel is a cornerstone of current therapy for acute myocardial infarction with shock. Guidelines are less clear about stenoses in non-infarcted–related arteries, but angioplasty can be beneficial if applied to high grade stenoses in vessels which supply a major portion of non-infarcted myocardium.

When emergent catheterization and possible angioplasty are not available, fibrinolytic therapy is recommended for ST-elevation myocardial infarction in patients with cardiogenic shock when there is no contraindication to fibrinolysis.

In the presence of extensive three-vessel coronary artery disease and post-infarction shock, emergency coronary artery bypass surgery is advisable in most instances. Time until revascularization is an important determinant of survival, in that mortality for patients undergoing coronary artery bypass

TABLE 11.4. Adrenergic receptor activity and other properties of sympathomimetic amines (Adapted from Kirklin et al., 2004).

	Alpha (peripheral vasoconstriction)	Beta$_1$ (cardiac contractility)	Beta$_2$ (peripheral vasoconstriction)	Chronotropic effect	Arrhythmia risk
Norepinephrine	++++	+++	0	+	+
Epinephrine	+++	+++++	+	++	+++
Dopamine[a]	++	+++	+	+	+
Dobutamine	0	+++	++	+	+
Isoproterenol	0	++++	+++	++++	++++
Phenylephrine	++++	0	0	0	0

[a] May cause renal arteriolar dilatation at low doses by stimulating dopaminergic receptors, moderate diuretic effect.

Table 11.5. Standard inotropic doses (Adapted from Kirklin et al., 2004).

Drug	Starting dose (μg/kg/min)	Dosing range (μg/kg/min)
Dopamine	2.5	2.5–20
Dobutamine	2.5	2.5–20
Milrinone	0.2–0.3	0.2–1.0
Epinephrine	0.025	0.025–0.1
Norepinephrine	0.025	0.025–0.1
Isoproterenol	0.025	0.025–0.1

grafting within 18 h of the onset of shock is about 40%, with a significant increase in mortality for longer intervals. ACC/AHA Guidelines indicate that emergency coronary bypass surgery should be considered in patients with cardiogenic shock who have significant left main or severe three vessel disease without major renal or pulmonary comorbidity.

Surgical Therapy for Complications of Acute Myocardial Infarction

In the setting of myocardial infarction complicated by rupture of the interventricular septum or rupture of a papillary muscle with severe mitral regurgitation, early emergent operation with mitral valve repair or replacement and/or surgical closure of the ventricular septal defect is mandatory. All such patients should be treated with intra-aortic balloon support prior to operation. These operations should be undertaken emergently, since the interval between diagnosis and operations is a critical determinant of survival.

Mechanical Circulatory Support

When shock persists despite standard measures including intra-aortic balloon support, inotropic agents and emergency angioplasty, more complex forms of mechanical circulatory support should be considered. Extra-corporeal membrane oxygenator (ECMO) support can be rapidly initiated in the intensive care unit setting via percutaneous femoral arterial and venous cannulation. This carries the advantage of rapid percutaneous cardiac support when intra-aortic balloon pumping and other standard interventions are not successful in reversing the shock syndrome. The major disadvantage of ECMO support is the lack of direct decompression of the left atrium with the potential for worsening pulmonary edema, particularly if diffuse capillary leakage (associated with the generalized inflammatory state) is accompanied by persistent elevation of left atrial pressure.

Other standard options for emergent mechanical circulatory support have been described in the earlier section on right ventricular mechanical support, and can provide right, left, or biventricular support. A variety of more chronic implantable volume-displacement or rotary ventricular assist devices are available, but paracorporeal devices are generally preferable in the setting of profound cardiogenic shock of rapid onset. More recently, European centers have reported experience with micro-axial blood pumps, such as the **Impella** (Abiomed – Danvers, MA), which can be inserted through the femoral artery or via a transthoracic approach.

Outcomes

When cardiogenic shock complicates myocardial infarction, the mortality remains excessive. Hospital mortality was approximately 90% during the 1970s and has improved in recent years with aggressive strategies for early reperfusion. Despite these improvements, current hospital mortality is still about 50%. The SHOCK study examined the hypothesis that emergency revascularization for cardiogenic shock due to myocardial infarction results in reduction of 30 day mortality compared with initial medical stabilization and delayed revascularization. Although 30 day mortality between the two groups was not statistically different, the survival at 6 and 12 months was significantly greater in the emergency revascularization group.

The benefit of early revascularization was most evident among patients less than 75 years of age. With an aggressive approach to the treatment of post infarction shock, aggressive early revascularization in patients under 75 years of age has reduced overall mortality to about 35%. The rewards of a strategy of aggressive early revascularization (in the cath lab or surgically) are underscored by the very favorable long-term survival of patients who survive to hospital discharge. Among shock patients who survive the first post-infarct year, annual mortality is less than 5%, similar to the general acute infarction population.

Based on the SHOCK trial, the ACC/AHA published a Class 1A recommendation for early invasive reperfusion in acute myocardial infarction complicated by cardiogenic shock for patients younger than 75 years of age; for patients over age 75 invasive intervention was recommended for those with good prior functional status. Current data suggests that an early aggressive invasive approach to myocardial support and revascularization should be the standard of care when acute myocardial infarction is complicated by cardiogenic shock. ACC/AHA Guidelines suggest that intra-aortic balloon pump support and/or ventricular assist devices should be considered for stabilization of deteriorating hemodynamics in preparation for emergent revascularization.

Selected Readings

Antman E, Anbe D, Armstrong P (2004) ACC/AHA guide-lines for the management of patients with ST-elevation myocardial infarction-executive summary. A report of the American College of Cardiology/American Heart Association Task Force on Practice Guidelines (Writing Committee to Revise the 1999 Guidelines for the Management of Patients with Acute Myocardial Infarction). J Am Coll Cardiol 44:671–719

Babaev A, Frederick P, Pasta D (2005) Trends in management and outcomes of patients with acute myocardial infarction complicated by cardiogenic shock. JAMA 294:448–454

Blume E, Duncan B (2006) Pediatric mechanical circulatory support in ISHLT monograph series. In: Frazier O, Kirklin J (eds) ISHLT monograph series: mechanical circulatory support. Elsevier, Philadelphia

Cinch J, Ryan T (1994) Current concepts: right ventricular infarction. N Engl J Med 330:1211–1217

Hochman J, Sleeper L, Webb J (1999) Should we emergently revascularize occluded coronaries for cardiogenic shock (SHOCK) investigators. Early revascularization in acute myocardial infarction complicated by cardiogenic shock. N Engl Med 341:625–634

Hollenberg S (2004) Recognition and treatment of cardio-genic shock. Semin Respir Crit Care Med 25:661–671

Holmes C, Walley K (2003) The evaluation and management of shock. Clin Chest Med 24:775–789

Kirklin J, Young J, McGiffin D (2004) Heart transplantation, 1st edn. Churchill Livingstone, New York

Mehta S, Eikelboom J, Natarajan M (2001) Impact of right ventricular involvement on mortality and morbidity in patients with inferior myocardial infarction. J Am Coll Cardiol 37:37–43

Sharp R, Gregory A, Mowdy M, Sirajuddin R (2004) Nesiritide for treatment of heart failure due to right ventricular dysfunction. Pharmacotherapy 24:1236–1240

Vida V, Mack R, Castaneda A (2005) The role of vasopressin in treating systemic inflammatory syndrome complicated by right ventricular failure. Cardiol Young 15:88–90

White H, Assmann S, Sanborn T (2005) Comparison of percutaneous coronary intervention and coronary artery bypass grafting after acute myocardial infarction complicated by cardiogenic shock: results from the Should We Emergently Revascularize Occluded Coronaries for Cardiogenic Shock (shock) trial. Circulation 112:1992–200

12
Nosocomial Pneumonia

Priya Sampathkumar

Pearls and Pitfalls

- Nosocomial pneumonia is the second most common nosoco-mial infection (after urinary tract infections) and represents the leading cause of nosocomial morbidity and mortality.
- Patients on mechanical ventilation have the highest risk of nosocomial pneumonia. Other patient populations at increased risk of pneumonia include burn, trauma, and cardiothoracic surgery patients.
- The term nosocomial pneumonia includes hospital-acquired pneumonia, ventilator-associated pneumonia, and *health care-associated pneumonia*. Health care-associated pneumonia is a newly described subset of nosocomial pneumonia that develops in patients who are not in the hospital at the time of onset but have had contact with the health care system up to 90 days prior to onset of pneumonia.
- Bacteria cause the majority of nosocomial pneumonia. Fungi are very uncommon causes of nosocomial pneumonia but can occur in immunocompromised hosts. Viruses, such as influenza, also may also cause nosocomial outbreaks.
- Aspiration of micro-organisms from the oropharynx or leakage of organisms around the cuff of the endotracheal tube is the primary mode of entry of bacteria into the lung. Pneumonia develops when host defenses against these organisms are overwhelmed.

K.I. Bland et al. (eds.), *Critical Care Surgery*,
DOI 10.1007/978-1-84996-378-7_12,
© Springer-Verlag London Limited 2011

- Early hospital-acquired pneumonia and early ventilator-associated pneumonia are likely to be caused by Pneumococcus, Hemophilus, and sensitive gram negative bacilli. In contrast, Pneumonia that occurs later in hospital stay is more likely to be due to multi-drug resistant organisms.
- Congestive heart failure, adult respiratory distress syndrome, and pulmonary contusions can mimic the appearance of pneumonia.
- Culture of lower respiratory tract secretions is the most useful diagnostic test in guiding therapy. Blood and pleural cultures may be helpful in selected situations.
- When treating pneumonia, treat early and aggressively with antibiotics. Target the most likely pathogens. Do not delay administration of antibiotics to obtain cultures.
- Re-evaluate when more data are available; focus pharmacologic therapy as soon as possible. Eight days of therapy is probably adequate for most nosocomial pneumonia *except* Pseudomonas pneumonia, where a minimum of 2 weeks is recommended.

Introduction

Nosocomial pneumonia has been defined traditionally as pneumonia that develops more than 48 h after admission to a health care facility, which was not present or developing at the time of admission.

This definition includes the subset of ventilator-associated pneumonia (VAP), which is defined as pneumonia developing >48 h after the onset of mechanical ventilation.

Recently, a new entity has been included in the nosocomial category: *health care-associated pneumonia* (HCAP), which refers to pneumonia developing in persons who have had contact with the health care system in one or more of the following ways:

1. Received home intravenous antibiotic therapy, chemotherapy, wound care, or hemodialysis within 30 days of onset of pneumonia

2. Resided in a long term care facility or nursing home within 30 days of onset of pneumonia
3. Hospitalized in an acute care hospital for 2 or more days within 90 days of the onset of pneumonia

The reason for the inclusion of HCAP under the nosocomial umbrella is that, although the onset may occur while the patient is in the community, HCAP is usually caused by antibiotic-resistant organisms similar to those seen in hospitalized patients. In addition, the severity, outcome, and recommended treatments resemble those for nosocomial pneumonia rather than for community-acquired pneumonia.

Thus nosocomial pneumonia now represents hospital-acquired pneumonia (HAP), ventilator-associated pneumonia (VAP), and HCAP.

Epidemiology

Nosocomial pneumonia is the second most common nosocomial infection in the United States and is associated with considerable mortality and morbidity. Pneumonia represents the leading cause of deaths due to nosocomial infections, increases hospital duration of stay by an average of 7–10 days, and results in an excess cost of more than US$40,000 per patient. Available data suggest that nosocomial pneumonia occurs at a rate of 5–10 cases per 1,000 hospital admissions, and the incidence increases 6-to 20-fold in mechanically ventilated patients. The risk of VAP is greater in surgical patients compared with medical patients; patients undergoing cardio-thoracic surgery have the highest risk.

The majority of nosocomial pneumonia is caused by bacteria. Occasionally, influenza and respiratory syncytial viruses cause outbreaks of nosocomial pneumonia in high risk patients such as children, the elderly, and immunosuppressed patients. Aspergillus pneumonia can occur in severely immunosuppressed patients, but overall, fungi and viruses are not important causes of nosocomial pneumonia.

Pathogenesis

For nosocomial pneumonia to occur, microbial pathogens first need to gain entry to the lower respiratory tract and then overwhelm normal host defense mechanisms.

Aspiration of micro-organisms from the **oropharynx** or leakage of organisms around the cuff of the endotracheal tube is the primary mode of entry of bacteria into the trachea. Inhalation of microorganisms from contaminated aerosols, hematogenous spread from bloodstream infections, or translocation from the gastrointestinal tract appear to be rare causes of pneumonia. Colonization of the lumen of the endotracheal tube with bacteria encased in a biofilm may play a role in the pathogenesis of VAP.

Factors that increase ease of entry of micro-organisms to the lower respiratory tract (intubation, bronchoscopy, supine positioning) and conditions that predispose to aspiration, such as sedation, altered mental status, tracheoesophageal fistula, gastro esophageal reflux, esophageal stricture, and neuromuscular disorders, increase the risk of pneumonia.

Factors that affect normal host defenses also promote pneumonia. Intubation, pain from surgical incisions, and paralysis impair the cough reflex which is the first line of defense against bacterial entry. Older age, malnutrition, metabolic acidosis, persistent hyperglycemia, and immunosuppressive medications impair both humoral and cell-mediated immunity and the ability of the lungs to clear aspirated micro-organisms. Prolonged antibiotic use and gastric acid suppression make it more likely that the oropharynx and upper airway will be colonized with resistant microorganisms that are more difficult for the body to fight off. Finally, lack of attention to practices of infection control could mean that health care workers carry multi-drug resistant organisms from one patient to another either via contaminated hands or equipment. The above risk factors can also be classified as patient-related, intervention-related, and infection control-related risk factors (Table 12.1). Most of the patient-related factors cannot be modified, whereas

TABLE 12.1. Risk factors for nosocomial pneumonia.

Patient-related factors

  Age >70 years

  Severe underlying illness

  Malnutrition

  Altered mental status

  Metabolic acidosis

  Hyperglycemia

Intervention-related factors

  Intubation and mechanical ventilation

  Immunosuppressive medications

  Gastric acid suppression

  Prolonged antibiotic use

  Supine positioning

  Surgical procedures on the chest and abdomen

  Sedation

Infection control factors

  Lack of appropriate hand hygiene by staff

  Contaminated respiratory care equipment

most of the risk factors in the other two categories can be modified successfully by an educational program.

Etiology: The time of onset of pneumonia is an important predictor of specific causative pathogens. Early onset VAP and HAP, defined as pneumonia occurring within 4 days of hospitalization or intubation usually carry a better prognosis and are more likely to be caused by antibiotic-sensitive bacteria. The organisms most commonly causing pneumonia in this group include *Streptococcus pneumoniae, Hemophilus influenzae,* and antibiotic-sensitive gram negative bacilli such as *Klebsiella* and *Enterobacter* species. Late onset HAP and

TABLE 12.2. Likely pathogens in early and late nosocomial pneumonia.

Condition	Most likely pathogens
Early VAP or HAP	• *Streptococcus Pneumoniae*
	• *Hemophilus influenzae*
	• Methicillin sensitive *Staphylococcus aureus (MSSA)*
	• Antibiotic-sensitive gram-negative bacilli
	Klebsiella pneumoniae
	Enterobacter species
Late VAP or HAP, HCAP[a]	*Pseudomonas aeruginosa*
	• *Resistant Klebsiella*
	• *Acinetobacter*
	• *Methicillin resistant staphylococcus aureus (MRSA)*
	• *Legionella pneumophila*

[a]Often multi-drug resistant organisms.

VAP, defined as pneumonia occurring after 5 or more days of hospitalization or intubation, tend to be caused by multi-drug resistant pathogens and are associated with poorer outcomes (see Table 12.2). Patients with HCAP who reside in long term care facilities or who have had recent exposure to antibiotics tend to have a spectrum of pathogens that resembles those seen in late onset HAP and VAP.

Pneumonia due to *Staphylococcus aureus* is more common in patients with diabetes, head trauma, patients in intensive care units and those with a recent history of influenza.

Nosocomial pneumonia due to fungi such as *Aspergillus fumigatus* may occur in solid organ or bone marrow/stem cell recipients or in otherwise severely immunocompromised patients. Nosocomial aspergillus infections should prompt a search for an environmental source of fungal spores, such as contaminated air ducts or the dust stirred up by hospital renovation or construction. *Candida* and Aspergillus species often colonize the airway of hospitalized patients; however, in the absence of severe immunosuppression, *those fungal species do not cause pneumonia* and do not require treatment. Influenza A can be the cause of nosocomial outbreaks during the influenza season (typically fall and winter). Respiratory syncytial virus (RSV) outbreaks are common in pediatric settings but can also occur in adult patients, especially those with hematologic malignancies.

Diagnosis

Diagnostic tests are important for two reasons: to decide whether pneumonia is the explanation for the patient's signs and symptoms and, second, to determine the etiologic pathogen. The best strategy to make the diagnosis of nosocomial pneumonia remains controversial. In most patients who are not intubated and who are immunocompetent, the diagnosis is made clinically based on presence of a new lung infiltrate plus clinical evidence that the infiltrate is of infectious origin. This evidence includes:

1. New onset of fever >38°C
2. Purulent sputum
3. Leukocytosis or leucopenia
4. Decrease in oxygenation

Although these criteria should raise suspicion of pneumonia, confirmation of the diagnosis of pneumonia is difficult, especially in intubated ICU patients, who may have many reasons to have one or more of these findings. Thus, using clinical criteria alone to diagnose VAP may result in over diagnosis and unnecessary use of antibiotics. Another drawback to using clinical criteria alone is that this method does not identify the etiologic agent.

The diagnosis of the etiologic agent requires generally a lower respiratory tract culture, which can include cultures of endotracheal aspirates, bronchoalveolar lavage (BAL) fluid, or protected specimen brush. Endotracheal cultures are easy to obtain and will usually contain the pathogens found by more invasive cultures. Colonization of the trachea, however, is very common, and a positive culture does not distinguish a pathogen from a colonizing organism. A tracheal aspirate is most useful when negative, as pneumonia is very unlikely in a patient with a negative culture of a tracheal aspirate provided that the patient has not had recent (in the last 72 h) change in antibiotics.

Quantitative cultures of lower respiratory tract specimens can also be used to guide therapy. For BAL fluid obtained either bronchoscopically or by blind suctioning, growth of more than 104 colony forming units (cfu)/ milliliter (ml) of fluid is suggestive of pneumonia. For specimens obtained using a protected specimen brush a threshold of 10^3 cfu/ml is used. The main problems with these approaches are that these tests are more invasive, are costly, have poor reproducibility, and require specialized laboratory and clinical skills. False negative results occur, especially in patients who have received antibiotic therapy before the sample is obtained; however, the specificity of these tests is greater than that of sputum/endotracheal aspirate cultures. When positive cultures above the diagnostic threshold are obtained by one of these techniques, they provide strong evidence that the patient has pneumonia with that organism.

Postmortem studies of VAP have demonstrated several characteristics pertinent to diagnostic testing. The process is often multifocal, frequently involving both lungs, and generally in the posterior and lower segments. VAP is often in multiple different phases of evolution at different sites at the same time. Prior antibiotic therapy can influence the number of bacteria found in lung tissue. The multifocal nature of VAP suggests that BAL and endotracheal aspirates can provide more representative samples than the protected specimen brush, which samples only a single bronchial segment. Because of the diffuse bilateral nature of VAP and predominance in dependent lung segments, "blind" BAL and use of a protected specimen brush may be as accurate as bronchoscopic sampling.

Many biologic markers have been studied in an effort to improve the diagnosis of pneumonia. Among critically ill patients, measurements of serum C-reactive protein and procalcitonin have not proven helpful in diagnosing pneumonia. Another biomarker-triggering receptor expressed on myeloid cells (TREM-1) appears promising. TREM-1 is a recently identified molecule involved in the inflammatory response to infection. Neutrophils and monocytes expressing high levels of TREM-1 infiltrate tissues infected with bacteria and fungi. TREM-1 is shed by the membrane of activated phagocytes and can be found in the soluble form (sTREM-1) in body fluids. Presence of sTREM-1 in BAL fluid can be detected rapidly using an immunoblot technique, is a strong predictor of pneumonia. This test may be helpful in distinguishing pulmonary infiltrates due to infectious causes from those from non-infectious causes, when it becomes commercially available.

Blood cultures are helpful when positive, but overall less than 25% of pneumonias are associated with bacteremia. Pleural fluid cultures are rarely necessary to make the diagnosis of pneumonia, but pleural fluid analysis may be helpful, in patients who do not respond to appropriate antibiotic therapy, to identify empyema which may need additional interventions such as a chest tube.

Treatment

Once the decision is made to initiate antibiotic therapy for nosocomial pneumonia, it is important to pick initial antimicrobial coverage that targets the most likely pathogens. Delayed or inappropriate antibiotic therapy is associated with poorer outcome. General principles of treatment are outlined in Table 12.3. The key decision in initial empiric antibiotic therapy is whether the patient has risk factors for multi-drug resistant organisms (MDR). These risk factors are summarized in Table 12.4. Patients deemed at risk of MDR organisms should receive broad spectrum coverage with antibiotics directed against these organisms. The specific choice of agents should be based on local patterns of antibiotic resistance and should also take into account antibiotics that the patient has received within the preceding 2 weeks. Whenever possible, antibiotics chosen for empiric treatment of the pneumonia should include

TABLE 12.3. Principles of antibiotic therapy for nosocomial pneumonia.

If patient at risk for multi-drug resistant organisms, use combination antibiotic therapy

Use intravenous antibiotics initially, switch to oral/enteral antibiotics in selected patients with good clinical response and functioning GI tract

If patient has had recent exposure to antibiotics, choose antibiotics for pneumonia from different antibiotic classes

Use local resistance patterns to guide choice of antibiotic

If patient received an initial appropriate regimen, short course therapy i.e. 7–8 days is adequate provided patient has a good clinical response and the pathogen being targeted is **not Pseudomonas**

TABLE 12.4. Risk factors for nosocomial pneumonia caused by multidrug resistant pathogens.

Immunosuppression

Current hospitalization of 5 days or more

Presence of known antibiotic resistance in the community or in the specific hospital unit

Risk factors for HCAP

- Chronic hemodialysis

- Residence in a long term care facility

- Receipt of home infusion therapy or wound care within 30 days of onset of pneumonia

- Hospitalization in an acute care facility for 2 or more days within 90 days of onset of pneumonia

antibiotics from drug classes to which the patient has not been exposed recently. For low risk patients, i.e., early onset VAP and HAP in patients without any of the risk factors for multi-drug resistant organisms, therapy should be targeted against common community-acquired pathogens in addition to *S. aureus* and *Enterobacter* species. An appropriate choice would be a respiratory quinolone (levofloxacin or moxifloxacin), a β-lactam/β-lactamase inhibitor combination (ampicillin-sulbactam), a non-pseudomonal cephalosporin (Ceftriaxone), or a limited spectrum carbapenem (Ertapenem).

Patients who have any risk factors for MDR pathogens should receive combination antibiotic therapy directed against these MDR organisms, including *Pseudomonas* and other resistant gram negatives. This combination should include an antipseudomonal cephalosporin (cefepime or ceftazidime) or carbepenem (Imipenem or Meropenem) or an anti-pseudomonal β-lactam/β-lactamase inhibitor combination (piperacillin/tazobactam) plus a second antipseudomonal drug - either a quinolone (ciprofloxacin or levofloxacin) or an aminoglycoside (amikacin, gentamicin or tobramycin). Because aminoglycosides have poor penetration into respiratory secretions and carry the risk of nephrotoxicity, especially in critically patients, we prefer a quinolone instead of an aminoglycoside whenever possible. Vancomycin or linezolid should be added to this regimen in patients known to be colonized with methicillin-resistant *S. aureus* (MRSA) and in hospital units with a high prevalence of MRSA (Fig. 12.1).

Initial therapy should be administered intravenously in all patients with a switch to oral/enteral therapy in selected patients who have a good clinical response and a functioning gastrointestinal tract. Dosing should be adjusted based on the patient's renal function. MDR strains of *Pseudomonas* and *Acinetobacter* resistant to all the commonly used antipseudomonal agents are being reported increasingly worldwide. Colistin, a drug in the polymyxin antibiotic class that fell out of favor several years ago because of its renal toxicity and the emergence of other effective antibiotics, is now regaining importance as the only current drug effective against these strains. Like the aminoglycosides, it is can be administered intravenously or as an aerosol. The aerosol route minimizes the risks of drug toxicity but generally should be used in addition to, not as a substitute for, a systemic agent.

Response to therapy: Clinical improvement usually becomes apparent after 48–72 h of onset of appropriate therapy. This improvement may be evidenced by decrease in white blood cell count and increased oxygenation with resolution of fever. Chest radiographs will not show improvement for several days and may actually get slightly worse in the first few days of treatment. All patients should be re-assessed at day 3 to

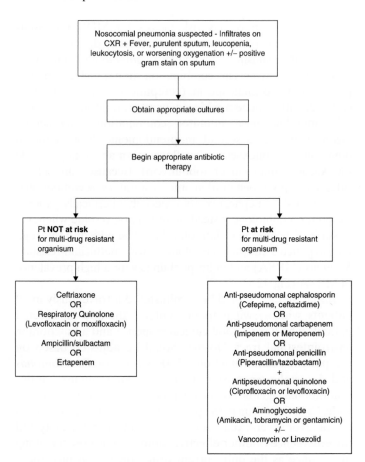

FIGURE 12.1. Treatment strategy for nosocomial pneumonia.

decide whether the initial diagnosis of nosocomial pneumonia was correct and to assess whether antibiotic therapy needs to be modified based on available culture data. For patients who are deteriorating or not responding to initial therapy, it may be necessary to broaden antibiotic coverage while simultaneously pursuing further diagnostic testing (Fig. 12.2), including repeating cultures of lower respiratory tract specimens and searching for an alternative site of infection, such as urinary tract or

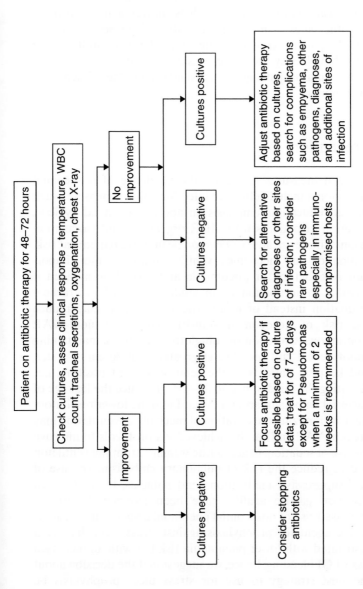

FIGURE 12.2. Re-evaluation 48–72 h after starting antibiotic therapy for suspected nosocomial pneumonia (Adapted from the American Thoracic Society and Infectious Diseases Society of America).

blood stream infection, surgical site infection, sinusitis, or a complication of pneumonia such as empyema. If the work up for other sites of infection/alternative diagnoses is negative and the patient remains febrile with pulmonary infiltrates, an open lung biopsy should be considered to diagnose infection with an unusual pathogen or a non infectious illness that mimics pneumonia.

Prevention

General measures to reduce the incidence of nosocomial pneumonia include effective infection control measures such as staff education, emphasis on appropriate hand hygiene, isolation of patients with MDR organisms, and vaccination against influenza and *S. pneumoniae* in those patients at risk. Intubation and mechanical ventilation are the most important risk factors for pneumonia and should be avoided if possible. If intubation is unavoidable, use of orotracheal intubation instead of nasotracheal intubation may reduce the risk of nosocomial sinusitis and subsequent VAP. Continuous aspiration of sub-glottic secretions, maintaining endotracheal cuff pressure at greater than 20 cm of water, and keeping patients in the semi-recumbent position, i.e., elevating the head of bed to 30–45° all reduce the leakage of bacterial pathogens around the cuff into the lower respiratory tract. Minimizing the duration of mechanical ventilation may prevent VAP and can be achieved via protocols to improve the use of sedation, to accelerate weaning from the ventilator, and to reduce the risk of pulmonary embolism. The use of acid-suppressive medications and antacids, both of which decrease gastric acidity, have been associated with an increased risk of nosocomial pneumonia. Sucralfate, an alternative agent for prophylaxis against stress ulcer, has been associated with lower pneumonia risk but with an increased risk of GI bleeding; hence, we suggest that the decision about the best strategy to use for stress ulcer prophylaxis be tailored to the individual patient.

Many institutions have adopted "bundles" by which several of these interventions are implemented together rather than individually. For instance, the VAP bundle promoted by the Institute for Healthcare Improvement in the US recommends all of the following interventions be implemented: the head of bed be raised to >30°, daily sedation holiday along with regular assessment of readiness for weaning, and prophylaxis against stress ulcer and deep vein thrombosis. The Hospital Infection Control Practices Advisory Committee (HICPAC) of the Centers for Disease Control and Prevention has also published comprehensive recommendations for the prevention of nosocomial pneumonia.

Selected Readings

Adair CG, Gorman SP, Feron BM, et al. (1999) Implications of endotracheal tube biofilm for ventilator-associated pneumonia. Int Care Med 25:1072–1076

Collard HR, Saint S, Matthay MA (2003) Prevention of ventilator-associated pneumonia: an evidence-based systematic review. Ann Int Med 138:494–501

Fagon JY, Chastre J, Wolff M, et al. (2000) Invasive and noninvasive strategies for management of suspected ventilator-associated pneumonia. A randomized trial. [Comment]. Ann Int Med 132:621–630

Gibot S, Cravoisy A, Levy B, et al. (2004) Soluble triggering receptor expressed on myeloid cells and the diagnosis of pneumonia. N Engl J Med 350:451–458

Guidelines for the management of adults with hospital-acquired, ventilator-associated, and healthcare-associated pneumonia (2005) American Thoracic Society and Infectious Diseases Society of America. Am J Resp Crit Care Med 171: 388–416

Hoffken G, Niederman MS (2002) Nosocomial pneumo¬nia: the importance of a de-escalating strategy for antibiotic treatment of pneumonia in the ICU. Chest 122:2183–2196

Kollef MH, Shorr A, Tabak YP, et al. (2005) Epidemiology and outcomes of health-care-associated pneumonia: results from a large US database of culture-positive pneumonia. Chest 128:3854–3862

Tablan OC, Anderson LJ, Besser R, et al. (2004) Guidelines for preventing health-care-associated pneumonia, 2003: recommendations of CDC and the Healthcare Infection Control Practices Advisory Committee. Morbidity & Mortality Weekly Report Recommendations & Reports 53(RR-3):1–36

13
Gastrointestinal Failure

Lena M. Napolitano

Pearls and Pitfalls

- Early aggressive fluid resuscitation is necessary to treat intestinal mucosal hypoperfusion associated with shock states to avoid non-occlusive mesenteric ischemia.
- Intestinal failure is defined as the reduction of functional gut mass below the minimal amount necessary for digestion and absorption adequate to satisfy the nutrient and fluid requirements for maintenance in adults or growth in children.
- Stress-related mucosal disease (SRMD) is multiple superficial erosions occurring in the proximal stomach involving superficial capillaries secondary to mucosal hypoperfusion.
- SRMD is commonly associated with UGI bleeding, but gastric perforations are rare.
- Mechanical ventilation and coagulopathy are the two greatest risk factors for SRMD.
- Acid suppression therapy should be instituted in all patients at risk for SRMD.
- Acute colonic pseudo-obstruction (ACPO) presents with features of large bowel obstruction, without a mechanical cause and is due to an imbalance in the autonomic control of colonic motility.

K.I. Bland et al. (eds.), *Critical Care Surgery*,
DOI 10.1007/978-1-84996-378-7_13,
© Springer-Verlag London Limited 2011

- Conservative therapy is the preferred initial management for ACPO while identifying and correcting potentially contributory metabolic, infectious, and pharmacologic factors.
- Active intervention for ACPO is indicated for patients deteriorating during initial management and for those with signs or symptoms of ischemia, perforation, significant pain, fever, leukocytosis, or respiratory compromise, and for those failing conservative therapy.
- Neostigmine is effective pharmacologic therapy in the majority of patients with ACPO but requires close cardiovascular monitoring. If this fails, colonic decompression with more invasive methods (colonoscopic, surgical, or radiologic), should be considered.
- ACPO patients with overt perforation or signs of peritonitis should be managed surgically.
- Intra-abdominal hypertension (intra-abdominal pressure ≥ 12 mmHg) and abdominal compartment syndrome (intra-abdominal pressure ≥ 20 mmHg) can result in intestinal mucosal hyperperfusion.
- Abdominal compartment syndrome is associated with new organ dysfunction or organ failure.
- Intra-abdominal pressure is measured by transduction of intravesicular urinary bladder pressure.
- In patients with acute abdominal pain out of proportion to physical findings, especially with a history of cardiovascular disease, acute intestinal ischemia should be suspected.
- Surgical treatment of acute intestinal ischemia due to arterial occlusion includes revascularization, resection of necrotic bowel, and when appropriate, a "second-look" operation 24 h after revascularization.
- Nonocclusive mesenteric ischemia is acute intestinal ischemia in the absence of fixed arterial obstruction and should be suspected in patients with low flow states or shock.

Gastrointestinal failure may manifest in a number of ways. Critically ill patients in intensive care units (ICUs) commonly develop gastrointestinal tract problems as a result of severe physiologic stress. Among the abnormalities observed in such patients are stress-related mucosal disease which may result in acute upper gastrointestinal hemorrhage, disturbances in gastrointestinal motility, mucosal edema related to hypoalbuminemia which may promote intestinal ileus and abdominal compartment syndrome, intestinal hypoperfusion and ischemia, infectious complications such as Clostridium difficile colitis, and ultimately short bowel syndrome and intestinal failure.

Stress-Related Mucosal Disease

Stress-related mucosal disease (SRMD) refers to the development of specific, discrete, gastric mucosal lesions in response to severe stress. Although more common in years past when resuscitation was not as well appreciated, SRMD can still occur and cause considerable morbidity and mortality in critically ill patients. Most (75–100%) critically ill patients demonstrate endoscopic evidence of mucosal damage within 24 h of admission to the ICU. Critically ill patients can manifest SRMD in a continuum ranging from superficial erosions that are usually diffuse to the development of stress ulcers, which are deeper mucosal lesions that tend to be more focal and are at higher risk for bleeding. The mortality rate from SRMD bleeding approaches 50%.

Clinically-evident bleeding – the presence of material with the appearance of coffee grounds in the nasogastric (NG) aspirate, guaiac-positive NG aspirate or stool, hematemesis, melena, or hematochezia – occurs in 5–25% of critically ill patients. *Clinically important* – bleeding affects 3–6% of patients, and it is more serious than clinically-evident bleeding, because it involves hemodynamic instability or the need for blood transfusion. Clinically important bleeding is defined as overt bleeding associated with a decrease in systolic blood pressure of more than 20 mmHg within 24 h after gastrointestinal (GI) bleeding, orthostatic increase in heart rate of 20 beats/min, and a decrease in systolic blood pressure of 10 mmHg when the patient assumes an upright position. Other criteria include a decrease in hemoglobin concentration of 2 g/dl and need for transfusion of two units of packed red blood cells within 24 h after bleeding; in addition, the failure of the hemoglobin concentration to increase after transfusion by at least the number of transfused units minus 2 g/dl is worrisome.

SRMD manifests as multiple superficial erosions occurring in the proximal stomach involving superficial capillaries secondary to mucosal hypoperfusion. SRMD is commonly associated with upper GI bleeding, but gastric perforations are rare. In contrast, peptic ulcer disease is manifest by discrete, deep erosions usually in the duodenum and is secondary to other reasons (drugs, H. pylori, hypersecretory states, etc.). In contrast to SRMD, perforation is common.

Acid suppression therapy should be instituted in all patients at risk for SRMD (Fig. 13.1). Gastric acid and pepsin are both necessary for the development of SRMD. Activated pepsin digests the gastric mucosal lining and is inactivated at a pH > 4. Therefore acid suppression therapy reduces gastric acid concentration, inactivates pepsin, and also stabilizes clot formation by facilitation of platelet activation and aggregation.

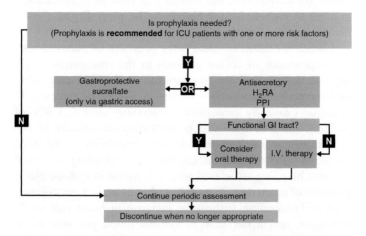

FIGURE 13.1. Algorithm for stress ulcer prophylaxis and prevention of stress-related mucosal disease (Adapted from ASHP Commission on Therapeutics, 1999. With permission).

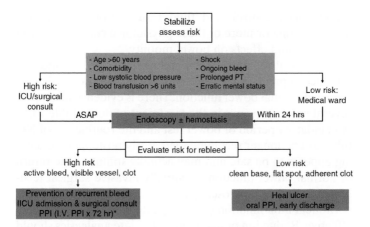

FIGURE 13.2. Algorithm for acute ulcer bleed.
Note: *role of selective second-look endoscopy is unclear (Adapted from Laine and Peterson, 1994. With permission. Copyright 1994 Massachusetts Medical Society. All rights reserved).

Risk factors for SRMD are many, but two strong independent risk factors consistently emerge, including respiratory failure requiring mechanical ventilation (odds ratio 15.6) and coagulopathy (odds ratio 4.3). Other risk factors for SRMD, including organ failure, sepsis, hypoperfusion states, traumatic brain injury, burns, and major surgery, also warrant SRMD prophylaxis. Furthermore, aggressive acid suppression therapy should be instituted promptly in any patient with acute upper GI hemorrhage (Fig. 13.2) in addition to endoscopy.

Intestinal Ileus

Intestinal ileus, the disturbance of bowel motility characterized by a lack of coordinated intestinal activity and a substantial overall reduction in peristalsis, is common in postoperative and critically ill patients. GI motility is coordinated by several physiologic mechanisms, including the autonomic nervous system, GI hormones, and inflammatory mediators. Anesthesia, surgery, pain control, and fluid resuscitation all alter the activity of one or more of these physiologic controls and can have profound effects on bowel motility.

Traditional regimens that emphasize bowel rest and NG tube decompression for the treatment of ileus do not hasten return of normal bowel function. There is evidence to support several newer concepts in the treatment of ileus (Table 13.1). A mandatory period of bowel rest and the routine use of NG tubes are no longer recommended. Early postoperative feeding appears to be safe and may actually stimulate the return of normal bowel function. Minimally invasive surgical techniques, including laparoscopy and other measures to decrease peritoneal inflammation such as gentle tissue handling, seem effective. Reduction or avoidance of opiate analgesics should be considered. The early institution of bowel regimens, including laxatives and rectal suppositories may be helpful, as is early ambulation. Excessive hydration should be avoided as intestinal edema may contribute to ileus. New pharmacologic agents, including m-receptor antagonists that selectively inhibit the effect of opioids on the gut or m-receptor agonists which could potentially produce effective analgesia without intestinal effects, are undergoing clinical investigation.

Acute Colonic Pseudo-Obstruction

Acute colonic pseudo-obstruction (ACPO) is characterized by massive colonic dilation in the absence of mechanical obstruction; synonyms include acute colonic ileus and Ogilvie's syndrome. Ischemia or perforation are the feared complications; spontaneous perforation has been reported in 3–15% of patients and carries a mortality of 50% or higher. The rate of perforation and/or ischemia increases rapidly with cecal diameters >10–12 cm and when the duration of distention exceeds 6 days. The pathogenesis is not completely understood but likely results from an imbalance in the autonomic regulation of colonic motor function; excessive parasympathetic suppression results in colonic atony and dilatation.

TABLE 13.1. Prevention and management of postoperative ileus (Adapted from Mattei and Rombeau, 2006. With kind permission of Springer Science and Business Media).

Category	Specific action	Physiologic effect
Pharmacologic	Minimize opiates	Decreases inhibitory effect of opioids
	Regional anesthesia techniques	
	(Prokinetic drugs)*	(Investigational)*
	(μ-agonists)*	
Inflammatory	Gentle handling of tissues	Decreases inflammation
	NSAIDs	
Hormonal	(Substance P antagonist)*	(Investigational)*
	(VIP antagonist)*	
Metabolic	Maintain electrolyte homeostasis	Decreases inhibitory effects of metabolic derangements
	Maintain acid-base balance	
	Maintain normothermia	
GI physiology	Early postoperative feedings	Stimulates bowel function
	Selective use of nasogastric tubes	
Neurologic	Thoracic epidural bupivacaine	Decreases sympathetic nervous activity
Psychologic	Educate patient regarding expectations of early discharge	Reduces anxiety

NSAID: nonsteroidal anti-inflammatory drug; VIP: vasointestinal polypeptide; IV: intravenous.

*Refers to investigational drugs under development that are used for their Prokinetic activity, ie improving intestinal movement and preventing intestinal ileus.

Early recognition and appropriate management are critical to minimizing morbidity and mortality. In evaluating a patient with signs or symptoms of suspected acute colonic dilation, mechanical obstruction must first be excluded, because surgical management otherwise may be required (Fig. 13.3). Although initial conservative management for mechanical obstruction overlays with the initial management of ACPO (e.g., nothing by mouth, intravenous fluids, nasogastric suction), the possibility of mechanical obstruction must always be considered, particularly if there is no response to conservative management. If there is any suspicion of mechanical obstruction, a water-soluble contrast enema of the rectum and distal colon should be obtained.

The causes of and predisposing factors are multiple (Table 13.2) and often more than one of these factors are present. Most commonly, this syndrome is associated with intraperitoneal or extra-peritoneal surgery, particularly pelvic and lumbar spine surgery. Based on LaPlace's law, increasing diameters accelerate the increase in tension within the colon wall. Although risk increases with expanding dimensions, there is only a poor association with absolute diameters. Some data suggest critical thresholds of 9 cm for the transverse colon and 12 cm for the cecum; however, many patients present with dimensions greater than this without sequelae. The acuity of onset and duration of persistent distention likely correlate more strongly with risk. Approximately 10% of patients have some degree of ischemia in the right colon at the time of colonoscopy. Spontaneous perforation has been estimated to occur in 3–15% of patients.

Conservative Therapy

The initial step in management of ACPO is to initiate therapy for potential contributing factors, including first evaluation for electrolyte and metabolic abnormalities (potassium, phosphorous, magnesium, calcium, and thyroid functions). Blood cultures and empiric antibiotics are indicated if sepsis is suspected clinically. Bowel rest with nasogastric decompression

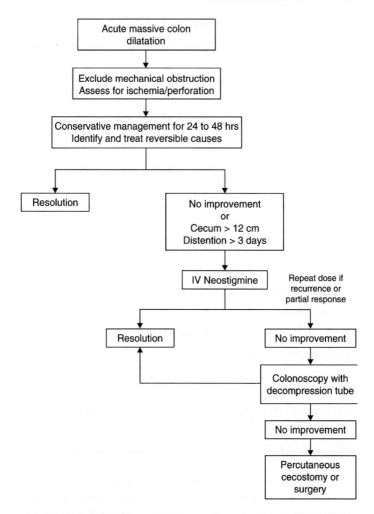

FIGURE 13.3. Algorithm for management of acute colonic distention (Reprinted from Saunders and Kimmey, 2005. With the permission of Blackwell Publishing).

should be initiated. Objective evidence of progress can be monitored radiographically by serial measurement of cecal diameter as often as every 8–12 h. Management includes discontinuation of narcotics, anticholinergic agents, and any

TABLE 13.2. Causes and predisposing factors associated with acute colonic pseudo-obstruction.

Postsurgical
Intra-abdominal operations
Other operative procedures
Lumbar/spinal and other orthopedic, gynecologic, urologic surgery
Renal transplantation
Trauma
Retroperitoneal trauma
Spinal cord injury
Medical
Age
Sepsis
Neurologic disorders
Hypothyroidism
Viral infection (herpes, varicella zoster)
Cardiac/respiratory disorders
Electrolyte imbalances (hypokalemia, hypocalcemia, hypomagnesemia)
Medications (narcotics, tricyclic anti-depressants, phenothiazides, anti-Parkinsonian drugs, anesthetic agents among others)
Renal insufficiency

other possible offending medications, exclusion of abdominal infection, mobilization out of bed if feasible, and appropriate medical and surgical management for significant concurrent illnesses. The direct benefits of any individual component of care are unknown, because these recommendations have not been studied as single interventions. A trial of conservative measures alone is appropriate in the subset of patients who lack significant abdominal pain, signs of peritonitis, and who have one or more potential underlying factors that are reversible.

Conservative management usually includes NG tube for gut decompression, aggressive use of optimal body positioning, and often, placement of a rectal tube with or without use of low-volume enemas. The prone position with hips elevated on a pillow or the knee chest position with the hips held high often aids the spontaneous evacuation of flatus. These positions should be alternated with right and left lateral decubitus positions regularly each hour, when feasible. When there is no pain and distention is not extreme (<12 cm), conservative measures can be used for 24–48 h before considering other medical or endoscopic intervention, particularly when reversible contributory factors are identified. During this interval, serial physical examinations for tenderness or signs of peritonitis should be performed and plain abdominal radiographs should be obtained every 8–12 h. The reported success of conservative management is variable, with rates from 20% to 92%.

Pharmacologic Therapy

The only consistently positive results have been with neostigmine. Neostigmine is an anticholinesterase, parasympathomimetic agent used for postoperative reversal of nondepolarizing neuromuscular blockade and in the treatment of myasthenia gravis and postoperative urinary retention. The belief that parasympathetic suppression, resulting in decreased colonic motility, plays a central role in ACPO is further supported by successful treatment of ACPO with intravenous neostigmine. Because such parasympathetic stimulation can induce bradycardia, asystole, hypotension, restlessness, seizures, tremor, miosis, bronchoconstriction, hyperperistalsis, nausea, vomiting, salivation, diarrhea, and sweating, administration must be accompanied by close cardiorespiratory monitoring. Toxicity is treated with atropine. Contraindications to use of neostigmine include known hypersensitivity and mechanical urinary or intestinal obstruction. Recent myocardial infarction, acidosis, asthma, bradycardia, peptic ulcer disease, and therapy with beta-blockers are relative contraindications to neostigmine therapy.

Endoscopic and Surgical Therapy

Approaches to mechanical decompression have included passage of decompression tubes under fluoroscopic guidance and colonoscopic decompression with or without placement of an indwelling, transanal decompression tube. Among the invasive therapeutic options, colonoscopic decompression is preferred, and success at the initial procedure, with or without tube placement varied from 61% to 78%, recurrence from 18% to 33%, almost all among patients without tube placement, and ultimate clinical success after one or more procedures was 73–88%. Complications occurred in 4% of patients and in-hospital, but unrelated, mortality rates were 13–32%. It remains unclear whether ischemia is an absolute contraindication to proceeding with decompression. The efficacy of colonoscopic decompression has not been established in randomized clinical trials. Also, perforations have been described in up to 3% of patients undergoing colonoscopic decompression.

Because operative management with colectomy or cecostomy carries greater morbidity than endoscopic decompression, it is therefore reserved for patients who fail endoscopic and pharmacologic efforts and for those in whom exploration of the peritoneal cavity might otherwise be indicated. Primary operative therapy is indicated for patients with predisposing intra-abdominal processes as well as those with suspected or evident free or contained perforation or peritonitis. Percutaneous cecostomy is also an option.

C. Difficile-Associated Disease

Clostridium difficile is a gram-positive, anaerobic, spore-forming bacillus that can cause pseudomembranous colitis and other *C. difficile*-associated diseases (CDAD). Two toxins, A and B, are involved in the pathogenesis of CDAD. Transmission occurs primarily in healthcare facilities, where exposure to antimicrobial drugs (the major risk factor for CDAD) and environmental contamination by *C. difficile* spores are more common.

About 3% of healthy adults and 20–40% of hospitalized patients are colonized with *C. difficile*, which in healthy persons is metabolically inactive in the spore form. The assumption is that perturbation of the competing flora promotes a conversion to vegetative forms that replicate and produce toxins. The characteristic clinical expression is watery diarrhea and cramps, and the characteristic pathologic finding is pseudomembranous colitis.

Early diagnosis and prompt aggressive treatment are critical in the management of CDAD (Fig. 13.4). The most common confirmatory study is an enzyme immunoassay for the *C. difficile* A and B toxins (sensitivity 93–100%, sensitivity 63–99%); results are available in 2–4 h. In severe cases, flexible sigmoidoscopy can provide an immediate diagnosis. Treatment consists of the prompt discontinuation of the implicated antimicrobial agent and the administration of oral metronidazole; for severely ill patients and those who do not have a prompt response to metronidazole, oral vancomycin should be considered. Prevention efforts should include fastidious use of barrier precautions, isolation of the patient, environmental cleaning with sporicidal agents active against *C. difficile*, and meticulous hand hygiene.

Both the rate and severity of CDAD is increasing in healthcare facilities worldwide. An increased severity of CDAD has been reported, with resulting admission to ICUs, need for colectomies, and deaths. A new epidemic strain of *C. difficile* has also been identified (BI/NAP1) which carries virulence properties and antibiotic resistance patterns of the European strain ribotype 027. These data have major implications for clinical care. Some institutions, in an effort to limit nosocomial spread, have instituted new practices. If a patient has clinically important diarrhea, he or she is started on oral metronidazole treatment immediately and placed on contact precautions, prior to obtaining the confirmatory test results.

These findings, in conjunction with the emergence of methicillin-resistant *Staphylococcus aureus* (MRSA) and

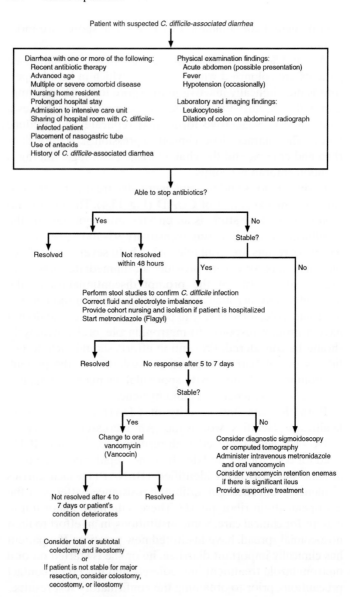

FIGURE 13.4. Algorithm for the treatment of C. difficile-associated diarrhea (Adapted from Viswanath and Griffiths, 1998. Reproduced from the BMJ Publishing Group. With permission).

vancomycin-resistant enterococcus (VRE), emphasize the need for all healthcare providers to prescribe antimicrobial agents judiciously and to comply with infection-control measures. The most important of these measures consists of meticulous hand hygiene. Increasing the use of alcohol-based waterless sanitizers has been an important method of increasing hand hygiene compliance among healthcare providers. It is important, however, to continue to encourage hand washing with soap and water when organisms that are resistant to alcohol-based cleaners, such as the potential spore-forming organism *C. difficile*, are identified in the local environment.

Intestinal Hypoperfusion and Ischemia

Ischemia of the intestine may manifest with different clinical features, each requiring a specific diagnosis and treatment approach. Patients with acute abdominal pain out of proportion to physical findings and who have a history of cardiovascular disease should be suspected of having acute intestinal ischemia.

Early identification and treatment of acute mesenteric ischemia is crucial to improve prognosis. Operative treatment of acute obstructive intestinal ischemia includes revascularization, resection of necrotic bowel, and when appropriate, a "second-look" operation 24 h after revascularization. Percutaneous interventions (including transcatheter lytic therapy, balloon angioplasty, and stenting) are appropriate in selected patients with acute intestinal ischemia caused by mechanical arterial obstructions. Patients so treated may still require laparotomy.

Acute intestinal ischemia sufficient to produce infarction also occurs in the absence of fixed arterial obstruction. Nonocclusive mesenteric ischemia (NOMI) should be suspected in patients with low flow states or shock, especially cardiogenic shock, who develop abdominal pain, in patients receiving vasoconstrictor agents, and after revascularization for intestinal ischemia caused by arterial obstruction. Treatment of the underlying shock state is the most important initial step in treatment of NOMI. Arteriography is indicated in patients suspected of NOMI whose condition does not improve rapidly with treatment of their underlying disease. Transcatheter administration of vasodilator medications into the area of vasospasm is indicated in patients with NOMI who do not respond to systemic supportive treatment and in those with intestinal ischemia due to cocaine or ergot poisoning. Laparotomy and resection of nonviable bowel is necessary in patients with NOMI who have persistent symptoms despite treatment.

Acute mesenteric ischemia remains a morbid condition with poor short-term and long-term survival rates. The contemporary management with revascularization with surgical or angiographic techniques, resection of non-viable bowel, and liberal use of second-look procedures can result in the early survival of two thirds of patients with embolisms and thrombosis. Variables independently associated with worse survival include age >60 years, bowel resection at first-look or second-look laparotomy and previous surgery.

Ischemic colitis, another form of intestinal ischemia, usually affects either just the right or just the left colon and may resolve spontaneously. Bowel rest, IV fluids, and antibiotics are the standard treatment. Initially, operative intervention is indicated for patients with peritonitis, massive bleeding, or fulminant colitis, or those who do not improve after 2–3 weeks of treatment, those evolving to sepsis, or those presenting late with colonic stricture or persistent chronic colitis. Chronic mesenteric ischemia has to be considered in elderly patients or those with risk factors presenting with postprandial abdominal pain and weight loss. Treatment may be performed either by operative revascularization or angioplasty with or without stent placement according to patient conditions and surgical risk.

Abdominal Compartment Syndrome

Intra-abdominal hypertension and abdominal compartment syndrome are being recognized increasingly in the critically ill. Intra-abdominal hypertension is defined by a sustained or repeated pathologic increase in intra-abdominal pressure ≥12 mmHg; it is at this pressure that reduction in intestinal microcirculatory blood flow occurs. Normal intra-abdominal pressure is approximately 5–7 mmHg in critically ill adults. Abdominal compartment syndrome is defined as a sustained intra-abdominal pressure ≥20 mmHg (with or without an abdominal perfusion pressure < 60 mmHg) that is associated with new organ dysfunction or failure.

Measurement of intra-abdominal pressure is accomplished by indirect means by transduction of intravesicular or "urinary bladder" pressure via the Foley catheter. Intra-abdominal pressure should be measured at end-expiration in the supine position after ensuring that abdominal muscle contractions are absent and with the transducer zeroed at the level of the mid-axillary line, and with a maximal instillation volume of 25 ml of sterile saline into the bladder.

Analogous to the widely accepted and clinically utilized concept of cerebral perfusion pressure, abdominal perfusion pressure is calculated as mean arterial pressure minus intra-abdominal pressure. Abdominal perfusion pressure has been proposed as a more accurate predictor of visceral perfusion and a potential endpoint for resuscitation. A target abdominal perfusion pressure of at least 60 mmHg correlates with improved survival from syndromes of increased intra-abdominal pressures.

Primary abdominal compartment syndrome is associated with injury or disease in the abdominopelvic region that frequently requires early surgical or interventional radiologic intervention. *Secondary abdominal compartment syndrome* refers to conditions that do not originate from the abdominopelvic region, and is commonly caused by massive volume resuscitation in a patient with no prior abdominal pathology, i.e., burn patient. *Recurrent abdominal compartment syndrome* (formerly termed tertiary abdominal compartment syndrome) refers to the condition in which abdominal compartment syndrome re-develops after treatment of primary or secondary abdominal compartment syndrome.

Prevention, early recognition, and treatment of abdominal compartment syndrome are of great importance in the prevention of intestinal mucosal hypoperfusion. If abdominal compartment syndrome is related to the development of tense ascites, paracentesis can be considered. In contrast, if abdominal compartment syndrome is related to intestinal and visceral edema, medical management with diuretic therapy or decompressive celiotomy must be considered. In patients at risk for abdominal compartment syndrome postoperatively, such as those where fascial closure would be difficult due to tension, delay in primary fascial closure using an open abdomen approach with delayed fascial closure may be considered. Serial monitoring of intra-abdominal pressure should be considered in all patients at risk.

Short Bowel Syndrome and Intestinal Failure

Intestinal failure can be defined as a decrease in functional gut mass below the minimal amount necessary for digestion and absorption adequate to satisfy the nutrient and fluid requirements for maintenance in adults or growth in children. Intestinal failure occurs when the body is unable to sustain its energy and fluid requirements without nutritional support, due to loss of functional small bowel. In developed countries, intestinal failure mainly includes individuals with the congenital or early onset of conditions requiring protracted or indefinite parenteral nutrition. Short bowel syndrome was the first commonly recognized cause of protracted intestinal failure.

The normal physiologic process of intestinal adaptation after extensive resection usually allows for recovery of sufficient intestinal function within weeks to months. Intestinal adaptation occurs when the remaining gut goes through functional and morphologic changes increasing its absorptive capacity. Factors such as intraluminal nutrients, gastrointestinal secretions, and GI hormones facilitate adaptation. Enteral feeds are a potent stimulant to adaptation and should be started as soon as the clinical situation permits. Some drugs thought to increase intestinal adaptation include glutamine, growth hormone, and glucagon like peptide-2, but there is a paucity of data to guide their use. During this time of intestinal adaptation, patients are sustained on parenteral nutrition. Non-transplant surgery, including small bowel tapering and lengthening to increase absorptive surface area, may allow weaning from parenteral nutrition in some patients. Congenital diseases of enterocyte development, such as microvillus inclusion disease or intestinal epithelial dysplasia, cause permanent intestinal failure for which no curative medical treatment is available. Severe and extensive motility disorders, such as total or subtotal intestinal aganglionosis (long segment Hirschsprung disease) or chronic intestinal pseudo-obstruction syndrome, may also cause permanent intestinal failure.

Prolonged intestinal failure due to short bowel syndrome occurs predictably after extensive intestinal resection and other problems (Table 13.3). Short bowel syndrome can be

TABLE 13.3. Etiology of short bowel syndrome (Adapted from Goulet and Ruemmele, 2006. With permission from the American Gastroenterological Association).

Prenatal	Neonatal	Postnatal
Atresia (unique or multiple)	Midgut volvulus (midgut or segmental)	Midgut volvulus
	Necrotizing enterocolitis	Arterial thrombosis
Midgut volvulus (malrotation)	Arterial thrombosis	Inflammatory bowel disease
Segmental volvulus	Venous thrombosis	Post-trauma resection
Abdominal wall defects		Extensive angioma
Gastroschisis > omphalocele		Non-occlusive mesenteric ischemia
Extensive Hirschsprung's disease		Multiple operations for intestinal obstruction
Apple peel syndrome		Multiple operations for intestinal and enterocutaneous fistulae

treated with bowel rehabilitation, parenteral nutrition, or intestinal transplantation. The mainstay of management is parenteral nutrition, which is costly and may be associated with the well-recognized problems of liver disease and catheter-related sepsis. Cessation of parenteral nutrition at the earliest possible stage is desirable, but for this, enteral autonomy has to be achieved first. When prolonged parenteral nutrition is unsustainable or associated with unacceptable side effects, small bowel transplantation should be considered as a treatment option (Fig. 13.5).

Studies on the outcome of short bowel syndrome show a clear correlation to intestinal anatomy, notably remaining jejuno-ileal length, presence of the ileocecal value, and the colon in continuity with the small bowel. Classification of patients with short bowel syndrome is therefore based on etiology and anatomic characteristics. Anatomic classification of short bowel syndrome, however, poses several difficulties because there is a marked variation in intestinal length in adults, and an even greater variation in children as a result of growth.

The normal length of the small bowel in adulthood has a mean of 550 cm with a wide range of 350–700 cm depending

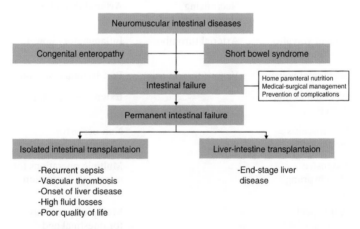

FIGURE 13.5. Management of intestinal failure (Reprinted from Goulet et al., 2004. With the permission of Lippincott Williams & Wilkins).

on race, body weight, and the size of the patient. It follows that exact anatomic quantification of the remnant intestinal length necessary to maintain intestinal autonomy is difficult. Individuals with healthy intestinal mucosa may be expected to regain or maintain intestinal autonomy with a jejuno-ileal length of 50–70 cm in the presence of an intact colon, or 150–200 cc in its absence. The determining factor remains the critical mass of residual functional intestinal absorptive epithelia. Therefore, there is a great need for a specific marker of functional epithelial mass and adaptive response, but no such markers have been widely identified.

New scientific advances, including the recent identification that a newly identified human protein (R-spondin1) increases dramatically the proliferation and growth of the small and large intestines in mice, are of great interest for the possible eventual treatment of intestinal disorders such as short bowel syndrome and intestinal failure.

Selected Readings

Abraham C, Cho JH (2005) Inducing intestinal growth. N Engl J Med 353(21):2297–2299

American Gastroenterological Association Clinical Practice and Practice Economics Committee (2000) AGA Technical Review on Intestinal Ischemia. Gastroenterology 118:954–968

ASHP Commission on Therapeutics (1999) ASHP report: stress ulcer prophylaxis. Am J Health Sys Pharm 56:347–379

Bartlett JG (2006) Narrative review: the new epidemic of Clostridium difficile-associated enteric disease. Ann Intern Med 145:758–764

Berman L, Carling T, Fitzgerald TN, Bell RL, Duffy AJ, Longo WE, Roberts KE (2008) Defining surgical therapy for pseudomembranous colitis with toxic megacolon. J Clin Gastroenterol 42(5):476–580

Byrn JC, Maun DC, Gingold DS, Baril DT, Ozao JJ, Divino CM (2008) Predictors of mortality after colectomy for fulminant Clostridium difficile colitis. Arch Surg 143(2):150–154; discussion 155

Fennerty MB (2002) Pathophysiology of the upper gastrointestinal tract in the critically ill patient: rationale for the therapeutic benefits of acid suppression. Crit Care Med 2002 (Suppl 30):S351–S355

Goulet O, Ruemmele F (2006) Causes and management of intestinal failure in children. Gastroenterology 130:S16–S28

Goulet O, Ruemmele F, Lacaille F, Colomb V (2004) Irreversible intestinal failure. J Pediatr Gastroenterol Nutr 38:250–269

Gupte GL, Beath SV, Kelly DA, et al. (2006) Current issues in the management of intestinal failure. Arch Dis Child 91:259–264

Hirsch AT, Haskal ZJ, Hertzer NR, et al. (2006) ACC/AHA 2005 Practice guidelines for the management of patients with peripheral arterial disease (lower extremity, renal, mesenteric, and abdominal aortic): a collaborative report from the American Association for Vascular Surgery/ Society for Vascular Surgery, Society for Cardiovascular Angiography and Interventions, Society for Vascular Medicine and biology, Society of Interventional Radiology, and the ACC/AHA Task Force on Practice Guidelines; endorsed by the American Association of Cardiovascular and Pulmonary Rehabilitation; national Heart, Lung and Blood Institute, Society for Vascular Nursing, Trans Atlantic Inter-Society Consensus; and Vascular Disease Foundation. Circulation 113:463–654

Laine L, Peterson WL (1994) Medical progress: bleeding peptic ulcer. N Engl J Med 331:717–727

Malbrain ML, Cheatham ML, Kirkpatrick A, et al. (2006) Results from the International Conference of Experts on Intra-abdominal Hypertension and Abdominal Compartment Syndrome. I. Definitions. Intensive Care Med 32:1722–1732

Mattei P, Rombeau JL (2006) Review of the pathophysiology and management of postoperative ileus. World J Surg 30:1382–1391

Saunders MD, Kimmey MB (2005) Systematic review: acute colonic pseudo-obstruction. Aliment Pharmacol Ther 15(22):917–925

Zerey M, Paton BL, Lincourt AE, Gersin KS, Kercher KW, Heniford BT (2007) The burden of Clostridium difficile in surgical patients in the United States. Surg Infect (Larchmt) 8(6):557–566

14
Diabetes Mellitus and Diabetes Insipidus

Martin D. Smith and Jacobus S. Vermaak

Pearls and Pitfalls

The Latin terms *diabetes* means "a siphon" or "passer through". *Insipidus* implies "tasteless", and *mellitus* "honeyed".

Diabetes Mellitus

- Diabetes mellitus (DM) is a systemic disease; the presenting surgical complaint should not overshadow the global approach needed in evaluating a patient with DM.
- The diabetic emergency can be challenging, and the surgical practitioner should have a clear approach to these very ill patients.
- Glycemic control (irrespective of whether the patient has diabetes mellitus or not) is important in the critically ill patient.
- Avoid complacency in patients thought to have only "mild" diabetes.
- Ultimately, there is no substitute for good patient education to decrease long-term diabetic complications.

K.I. Bland et al. (eds.), *Critical Care Surgery*,
DOI 10.1007/978-1-84996-378-7_14,
© Springer-Verlag London Limited 2011

Diabetes Insipidus

- The clinician must make the distinction from other causes of polyuria.
- Central and nephrogenic diabetes insipidus (DI) have different clinical and management implications.
- Prevention of hypernatremic dehydration is of critical importance, particularly in patients unable to regulate their own fluid requirements (e.g. the critically ill, the comatose patient, and small infants).

Diabetes Mellitus

Diabetes mellitus (DM) is the most frequent endocrine abnormality encountered by the surgeon. An increased serum glucose concentration is encountered commonly in surgical practice. This finding has ramifications for both the diabetic and non-diabetic patient. DM can present to the surgeon as either:

1. Co-morbidity, e.g. the diabetic patient requiring an inguinal hernia repair
2. A primary surgical pathology:

    (a) Acute complications of diabetes mellitus (e.g. diabetic ketoacidosis (DKA) presenting with a surgical abdomen)
    (b) Chronic complications of diabetes mellitus (e.g. diabetic foot)

Diagnosis

Non-diabetic patients often demonstrate an increased serum glucose concentration during periods of physiologic stress due to activation of the hypothalamic pituitary axis, catecholamine release, and peripheral resistance to insulin. Anxiety to venipuncture in itself can increase the serum glucose concentration. It is thus clear that, although an increased glucose concentration is specific for the diagnosis of DM, it lacks sensitivity.

Timely analysis of the serum glucose specimen is essential as continual glycolysis in the cells renders unpredictably lower values. Whole blood glucose values are up to 15% lower and arterial values up to 7% higher than corresponding plasma values. Capillary whole blood, used in bedside monitoring and serum plasma glucose levels are nearly equivalent. For the purposes of the chapter, we will refer to serum glucose levels only.

Diabetes Mellitus can be diagnosed easily in patients with unequivocal hyperglycemia and the classic DM symptoms of polydipsia, polyuria, DKA, hyperosmolar non-ketotic diabetic coma (HONK), or complications of prolonged exposure to hyperglycemia, with resultant end-organ damage.

For patients without classic symptoms but in whom DM is suspected, an oral glucose tolerance test (OGTT) should be performed: 75 g of anhydrous glucose is given orally (in children 1.75 g/kg up to a dose of 75 g). Glucose values are taken before glucose administration (after an overnight fast of 8–14h) and 2h after the glucose load. See Table 14.1 for diagnostic values. We recommend that the diagnosis of diabetes mellitus never be made on a single serum glucose value in the asymptomatic patient.

TABLE 14.1. Serum glucose values for the diagnosis of diabetes mellitus and glucose intolerance (Adapted from the WHO recommendations (World Health Organization, 1985).

	Serum glucose level mmol/l (mg/dl)
Diabetes mellitus	
Fasting level, *or*	Gluc ≥7 (126 mg/dl)
2 h post glucose load, *or both*	Gluc ≥11.1 (200 mg/dl)
Impaired glucose tolerance	
Fasting level, *and*	Gluc <7.0 (126 mg/dl)
2 h post glucose load	7.8 (140) ≤ Gluc < 11.1 (200 mg/dl)

When the diabetic patient presents to the surgeon, the following needs consideration:

1. The type or classification of DM
2. Duration of exposure to hyperglycemia
3. Systemic effects of DM
4. Diabetic emergencies
5. Long-term management of the patient

Classification of DM

Some clinicians use the terms "type 1" DM and "type 2" DM as synonyms for insulin-dependent diabetes mellitus (IDDM) and non-insulin-dependent diabetes mellitus (NIDDM) respectively. It is correct to reserve the term "type 1" diabetes for the immune-mediated DM, and the term "type 2" for the non-immune-mediated DM.

Diabetes mellitus can be classified as follows:

Primary

1. *Type 1 DM* may be diagnosed at anyage but is most frequently diagnosed before the age of 30. The primary pathology is the autoimmune destruction of pancreatic beta-cells. Patients are prone to develop DKA and usually will require insulin for glycemic control.
2. *Type 2 DM* is more common and is diagnosed usually after the age of 40 in obese patients due to a decreased peripheral utilization of insulin with insulin "resistance." Patients are more prone to develop hyperosmolar, non-ketotic diabetic coma, and the majority of patients can be controlled on oral hypoglycemic agents. Some patients may have to be controlled on insulin if oral hypoglycemic agents are unsuccessful.
3. MODY (maturity-onset diabetes of young people) is a "non-insulin-dependent diabetes" that has an atypical clinical pattern in that it presents in young adults who are frequently not obese. There is an autosomal dominant inheritance.

Secondary

1. Pancreatic disease. This form of acquired diabetes includes conditions that affect the exocrine pancreas: chronic pancreatitis, pancreatectomy, cystic fibrosis, and pancreatic trauma. Extensive destruction of the pancreas must occur before the reduction in beta cell mass is sufficient enough to ensure diabetes. The exception is pancreatic malignancy, notably adenocarcinoma, which is often associated with new onset diabetes. Unfortunately, this condition cannot be used as a screening test for pancreatic cancer because of its non-specificity and decreased sensitivity.
2. Medication (N-3-pyridylmethyl-N'-p-nitrophenyl urea, the rodenticide Vacor, which is irreversibly cytotoxic to beta cells).
3. Genetic syndromes (e.g. the lipodystrophies).
4. Hormonal induced (e.g. Cushing's disease and pheochromocytoma).
5. Pregnancy (gestational diabetes).

Glucose intolerance itself is not formally classified as diabetes but is predictive for progression to established diabetes.

Duration of DM

Preoperative evaluation of glucose control is important, because prolonged exposure to hyperglycemia poses a risk of serious systemic complications. Especially important is identification of a "brittle diabetic" with erratic glucose control. Certain proteins, notably the B-chain of hemoglobin A and albumin, become glycated. The glycated fraction hemoglobin (measured as HBA1c) normally represents less than 6% of the total hemoglobin; an abnormally high value provides a representation of glucose control over the preceding 3 months. Similarly, glycated albumin (measured as fructosamine) retains the half-life of albumin (21 days) and can provide an estimate of glycemic control for the preceding 3 weeks.

The Systemic Effects of DM

Retinopathy

Most diabetic patients have some degree of retinopathy which is dependent on the duration of disease. Retinopathy is a sensitive predictor of end organ damage. Progressive changes can be seen on fundoscopy. Initially microaneurysms, dot and blot hemorrhages and hard exudates (collectively referred to as "background retinopathy", or nonproliferative retinopathy) occur between 3 and 5 years after the onset of diabetes. When abnormal vessels become occluded, cotton wool exudates are seen (preproliferative retinopathy). The ischemic response stimulates neovascularization (proliferative retinopathy) and then finally fibroproliferative changes which can lead to retinal traction and detachment.

Nephropathy

About a third of patients with diabetes will develop nephropathy. Patients with IDDM are more likely to develop nephropathy than those with NIDDM. The first clinically detectable sign of diabetic nephropathy is microalbuminuria (30–300 mg of albumin/24 h). Microalbuminuria is not detectable by standard urine reagent sticks which generally only detect proteinuria greater than 550 mg/dl. Microalbuminuria is a strong predictor for progression to nephrotic syndrome, hypertension, and eventual end-stage renal disease. Interestingly, persistent microalbuminuria also appears to be predictive for cardiovascular mortality in DM.

Asymmetrical, sensory, peripheral neuropathy is the most common disease pattern. A minority of patients have a painful, peripheral neuropathy. The motor nerves may be involved with focal neuropathies, mononeuritis multiplex, and radiculopathies. Autonomic neuropathy may affect vascular tone, cardiac function, gastric motility, bladder emptying, and erectile function. The autonomic neuropathy may present as a resting tachycardia, abnormal diaphoresis, or postural hypotension alone. Autonomic neuropathy is important to the anesthesiologist, but it affects anesthesia due to increased hemodynamic instability and aspiration due to gastroparesis.

Macrovascular Complications

Accelerated atherosclerotic disease of large vessels is responsible for major morbidity and mortality in DM. More than 75% of diabetic patients will succumb due to complications of diabetic vascular disease, such as coronary artery disease, hypertensive disease, stroke, heart failure, and peripheral vascular disease. In addition, 7% of deaths are attributable to renal failure. The reason why diabetic patients experience accelerated atherosclerosis is unclear, but glycation of lipoproteins and increased platelet adhesion through various means are some of the proposed mechanisms.

The "diabetic foot" is the culmination of multiple systemic effects of diabetes. Peripheral neuropathy results in loss of sensation and altered foot architecture (secondary to motor neuropathy) which increases the risk of unrecognized trauma. Chronic ulceration and poor wound healing is perpetuated by the increased risk of infection, poor nutritional status, and deprived blood. In addition, the hyperglycemia is associated with impaired leukocyte function: chemotaxis, phagocytic capabilities, intracellular killing, and abnormal respiratory burst and superoxide formation. Uncontrolled diabetes puts the patient into a state of malnutrition by producing a relative state of constant catabolism, because the modulating effect of insulin on proteolysis, lipolysis, and glycogenolysis is lost. Because no convincing evidence supports the concept that malnourishment causes diabetes, the term "malnutrition-related diabetes" (MRDM) is obsolete. A previous subtype of MRDM, Fibrocalculous Pancreatic Diabetes (FCDM) is now classified as a disease of the exocrine pancreas which leads to DM.

In the preoperative evaluation of the diabetic patient a thorough investigation is required to identify the above complications.

Diabetic Emergencies

Medical Emergencies

1. Diabetic ketoacidosis (DKA). DKA occurs due to the loss of the modulating effect of insulin on free fatty acid metabolism. The result is ketone-formation and severe fluid deficit. The patient has altered consciousness, ketotic breath, and acidotic breathing. Metabolically, patients have hyperglycemia, a metabolic acidosis, and frequently severe pre-renal azotemia and dehydration secondary to the osmotic diuresis of the extreme hyperglycemia. Serum amylase activity is commonly increased, but it is rare to have concurrent pancreatitis. Even though the serum potassium is in the normal range (3.5–4.5 mEq/l) because of the acidosis, the total body potassium is severely depleted and should be replaced actively despite an ostensibly normal serum concentration. A septic focus is often present and should be sought actively: e.g. pneumonia, urinary tract infection, etc.

2. Hyperosmolar non-ketotic diabetic coma (HONK). HONK occurs in diabetic patients secondary to the dehydration associated with hyperglycemic osmotic diuresis. This serious condition carries a mortality in excess of 50%. In contrast to DKA, these patients are more prone to seizures, have higher plasma glucose levels (frequently more than 40 mmol/l), and have an even larger fluid deficit. Serum osmolality commonly exceeds 350 mOsm/kg.

3. Other medical emergencies also need consideration, notably the diabetic patient's propensity for "silent" myocardial infarction; diabetic patients might not experience pain or are more prone to present with atypical pain when having a myocardial infarction.

Surgical Emergencies

An aggressive approach must be adopted for the management of diabetic sepsis. Glycemic control may not be achieved if the source of sepsis is not addressed. Life-threatening surgical infections must always be excluded in the diabetic who presents in DKA, specifically wet gangrene, necrotizing fasciitis, emphysematous cholecystitis, and mucormycosis.

Pre-operative Preparation

Elective Procedures (The Diabetic Patient Admitted for Unrelated Pathology)

The approach to these patients includes assessment of recent glycemic control and the systemic complications of diabetes. Patients should be counselled about of the effects of long-term glycemic exposure with regard to nutritional status, surgical fitness, and wound healing.

Patients on oral hypoglycemic agents with good glycemic control may not have to stop their medication for minor procedures. When major operations are planned, oral hypoglycemic agents with a long duration of action should be stopped 24 h prior to operation, while those with short duration of action should be discontinued on the day of operation. Long-acting insulin is replaced by short-acting insulin. The patient should then be placed on an insulin sliding scale and 5% dextrose/water infusion to prevent hypoglycemia. The exact protocol should be determined by unit policy and the specific needs of the patient. Whether intermittent insulin administration or continuous infusions are used depends largely on the intensity of the available nursing care (intensive care vs. a normal day care ward). Although preferred, a continuous insulin infusion requires close supervision, and hypoglycemia has dire consequences. Regular glucose monitoring is essential during the procedure. Oral hypoglycemic agents may be restarted with normalization of enteric feeding. In the postoperative period, patients may become insulin-resistant temporarily, and the oral hypoglycemic agents might not attain good glycemic control. Strong evidence exists with regard to the benefits of tight glucose control in the postoperative period. The benefits relate mainly to a decrease in infection-related complications and a modulating effect on the release of inflammatory mediators.

Emergency Procedures

With rare exception, no patient with DKA or HONK should be taken directly to the operating room. The physiologic stress of operation coupled with the immense fluid deficit and metabolic derangement carry a high mortality rate. While it is true that glycemic control is difficult in a diabetic patient with a septic focus, one should address the metabolic derangement and demonstrate a trend toward reversal before undertaking an operation. Insulin and fluids are continued during the procedure.

Although DKA can mimic an acute abdomen, an intraabdominal septic focus (such as appendicitis) can initiate the ketotic process. The surgeon's priority should be to correct the underlying metabolic derangement and employ noninvasive diagnostic tests to aid the diagnosis. At the other end of the spectrum, diabetic patients may not present with classic signs of peritonitis due to the neuropathy.

The Management of DKA

The patient should be admitted to a high care facility. The mainstay of management is to administer insulin to arrest ketogenesis with replacement of fluid and potassium loss. Infusion of large volumes of crystalloid is recommended. Potassium is replaced expectantly, even if serum values are normal. Insulin should preferably be administered intravenously, but intramuscular administration can be considered while venous access is being established. Although phosphate levels also decrease during resuscitation, it is recommended to treat this expectantly. The use of sodium bicarbonate is not recommended unless the pH is less than 6.9 because of side effects such as hypernatremia, hypokalemia, and a relative cerebrospinal fluid acidosis-despite an increase in serum pH. The end-point of the intervention is not normalization of serum glucose level but rather normalization of ketotic acidosis, because the patient can still be in DKA with a normal serum glucose concentration. When the serum glucose approaches levels less than 15 mmol/l, fluid resuscitation should continue, but with 5% dextrose water to counteract the hypoglycemic effects of the insulin infusion. Although the endpoint of treatment is reversal of the ketoacidosis, the risk-benefit ratio needs to be considered seriously for the patient who requires an urgent operative procedure.

Glycemic Control in the Critically Ill Patient

New onset hyperglycemia is common in critically ill patients, and tight glucose control is recommended, because hyperglycemia in critically ill patients has been shown to be an independent risk factor for poor outcome. Whether the beneficial effects of tight glucose control come from the actual administration of insulin or from the normalization of glycemia remains unknown. Several groups have postulated that insulin per se could be responsible for the benefits observed through its anabolic effects.

Long-Term Management of the Diabetic Patient

A multidisciplinary approach is essential; involvement of the primary care practitioner, the family, a dietician, the podiatrist, and specialist physicians are essential. Weight control and dietary measures might be the only requirements for glycemic control in the patient with NIDDM. Cessation of smoking and regular exercise should be encouraged. The family should be involved and be informed of the warning signs of hypoglycemia. The patient should wear a bracelet identifying him or her as a diabetic. Education is indispensable, and counseling at every encounter with a health care worker is essential.

Due to the high sensitivity of a fasting plasma glucose level, screening programs can be implemented to avoid the long-term complications of diabetes mellitus.

Diabetes Insipidus

Diabetes insipidus (DI) is a collective term used to describe impairment of renal conservation of water related either to impaired vasopressin secretion or to an abnormal renal response to vasopressin. Diabetes insipidus that develops due to decreased vasopressin secretion from the neurohypophysis is referred to as "central DI" and is usually the consequence of head trauma or a post-operative effect of neurosurgical procedures. A decrease in the renal response to vasopressin is referred to as "nephrogenic DI" related to nephropathy. See Table 14.2.

The Diagnosis of DI

In the absence of other factors, large volumes of dilute urine, as much as 3–6 ml/kg/day, with an osmolality of less than 200 mOsm/kg, is virtually diagnostic. As a response to polydipsia, conscious patients are able to maintain their own fluid balance. In contrast, in the intensive care scenario, where the patient's autonomy for self-regulation of fluid balance is limited, or when managing small infants who are unable to communicate thirst, prevention of hypernatremic dehydration is a priority.

The diagnosis of DI is established when a patient is unable to reduce their urine output and increase urine osmolality after a period of controlled fluid deprivation. Central versus nephrogenic DI can be distinguished by the patient's ability to increase urine osmolality after the administration of DDAVP (1-deamino-8-D-arginine vasopressin) in central DI.

Diabetes insipidus needs to be differentiated from other causes of polyuria, such as primary polydipsia, metabolic disease (diabetes mellitus, hypercalcemia), systemic illness (myeloma, sickle cell disease, resolving acute tubular necrosis), and medications (diuretics, etc.).

TABLE 14.2. Comparing central and nephrogenic diabetes insipidus (DI).

	Central DI	Nephrogenic DI
Pathophysiology	↓Circulating vasopressin	↓Renal response to vasopressin
Etiology	Head injury	Polycystic kidney
	Hypothalamic neoplasms	Nephrotic syndrome
	Cerebral aneurysms	Amyloidosis
	Stroke	Sjögren's syndrome
	Meningitis	Myeloma
	Idiopathic	Lithium
		Normal aging process
Genetics	Autosomal dominant	X-linked
		Autosomal recessive
Management	Adequate fluid management	Adequate fluid management
	Address the cause, if possible	Address the cause, if possible
	DDAVP	Indomethacin
	Vasopressin	Amiloride
	Clofibrate	Thiazide diuretics
	Carbamazepine	

Physiology and Pharmacology of DI

Vasopressin is synthesized in the supraoptic and paraventricular nuclei of the hypothalamus and stored in the posterior lobe of the pituitary gland. Circulating vasopressin binds to vasopressin receptors found in vascular tree, many areas of the central nervous system, the adrenal glands, and platelets. The drug vasopressin has an enhanced clinical effect on V1 receptors causing vasoconstriction, platelet aggregation, and decreased

splanchnic perfusion and has benefit in the resuscitative sce-
narios of cardiac arrest and upper gastrointestinal bleeds. V_2
receptors are concentrated in the renal collecting ducts.
Stimulating V_2 receptors allow water channel proteins, called
aquaporins, to increase water extraction from the renal collecting ducts in order to concentrate urine. The synthetic ana-
logue of vasopressin 1-deamino-8-D-arginine vasopressin
(DDAVP, or desmopressin) can be administered intravenously
or intranasally with equal effect and differs from vasopressin
in being longer-acting and having its clinical effect primarily
on V_2 receptors without producing vasoconstriction. DDAVP
stimulates endothelial cells to release Factor VIII, a property
with clinical application in Hemophilia A and Von Willebrand's
disease.

Treatment of DI

Both types of diabetes insipidus need attention to fluid
management and especially so when the patient's autonomy
is diminished. Prevention of hypernatremic dehydration by
consciously increasing fluid intake is essential. The underlying
cause needs to be addressed.

Central DI: The abnormality with central DI is a decreased
circulating vasopressin, and thus, treatment with DDAVP is
appropriate. Vasopressin, however, has side-effects, such as
vasoconstriction, reduced splanchnic perfusion, and platelet
aggregation, as well as ACTH release and increased glycogenolysis, each of which limits its potential usefulness in central
DI. Other medications to potentiate the effects of a low circulating endogenous vasopressin level can also be considered,
including clofibrate, used in hyperlipidemia, carbamazepine,
an anti-epileptic drug, and chlorpropamide, a dangerous sul-
fonylurea with a long half-life and associated prolonged hypoglycemia; this latter drug is generally not recommended.

Nephrogenic DI: Certain medications can be used as an
adjunct to fluid management to increase the renal response
to circulating vasopressin, including NSAIDs, in particular,
indomethacin, which seems to enhance the antidiuretic

response to vasopressin, and amiloride, useful in lithium-induced nephrogenic DI. Amiloride blocks the uptake of lithium by the sodium channels in the collecting ducts. Ironically, a thiazide diuretic can be effective for the management of nephrogenic DI, although its mechanism of action in DI is uncertain.

The management challenge in DI relates to controlling the patients fluid and electrolyte status, particularly in the intensive care setting. Prognosis is related to the underlying cause, and medication can be used to decrease the morbidity associated with polyuria and polydipsia.

Selected Readings

Butler SO, Btaiche IF, Alaniz C (2005) Relationship between hyperglycemia and infection in critically ill patients. Pharmacotherapy 25:963–976

Coursin DB, Connery LE, Ketzler JT (2004) Perioperative diabetic and hyperglycaemic management issues. Crit CareMed 32(Suppl): S116–S125

The Expert Committee on the Diagnosis and Classification of Diabetes Mellitus (1997) Report of the Expert Committee on the Diagnosis and Classification of Diabetes Mellitus. Diabetes Care 20:1183–1197

Falanga V (2005)Wound healing and its impairment in the diabetic foot. Lancet 366:1736–1743

Jackson EK (1996) Vasopressin and other agents affecting renal conservation of water. In: Hardman JG, Limbird LE, Molinoff PB, et al. (eds) Goodman and Gilman's the pharmacological basis of therapeutics, 9th edn. McGraw-Hill, NewYork, pp 715–731

Montori VM, Bistrian BR, McMahon MM (2002) Hyperglycemia in acutely ill patients. JAMA 288:2167–2169

Nathan DM (1993) Long-term complications of diabetes mellitus. N Engl J Med 328:1676–1685

World Health Organization (1985) Diabetes mellitus: report of a WHO Study Group. Technical Report Series 727. WHO, Geneva

Index